Healthy
Stories

*Dedicated to the limited
number of Public Health
Servants and to the vast
number of those who serve
Public Health,*

*And to the Editors' and
Authors' families.*

ISBN: 978-0-615-29169-7
Copyright 2009.
Printed on recycled paper.
Printed in the United States of America.

Healthy
Stories

America's Award-Winning
Public Health Story Book

EDITOR-IN-CHIEF
Morton Laitner

SENIOR EDITORS
Amy Tejirian
Tracie L. Dickerson

ASSOCIATE EDITORS
Roland R. Pierre
Ninfa Urdaneta
J.D. Shingles
Heather Beaton
Frederick Villari

CIRCULATION MANAGERS
John Holmes, North Florida
Lori Jordahl, South Florida

ASSISTANT TO EDITORS
Gertrude Pendleton

Our Mission

Promoting and protecting health through stories.

Our Vision

Creating a world-class, public health short story book.

Our Goals

To delight our readers
through laughter, tears and thought;

On how their health and health departments
affect their well-being;

While coaching booklovers on the art of story-telling
as the principal method to get their message heard,
understood and remembered;

Inspiring readers to write their health experiences for others
to make a personal connection with their own lives;

While always remembering not to take ourselves too seriously
and that humorous stories make the best medicines.

Stories

FOREWORD

From the Administrator of the Miami-Dade County Health Department

As *Healthy Stories* celebrates its third edition, I am proud the book received a Model Practice Award from the National Association of County and City Health Officials (NACCHO) as an innovative program which educates the general population and more, specifically, health workers in the field of public health. Story-telling is one of our best practices. *Healthy Stories* continues to strengthen our Health Department and advance our mission-"To promote and protect the health of community through prevention and preparedness today, for a healthier tomorrow." Our stories motivated our readers to take charge of their health and compeled them to help others through charitable contributions.

These stories are a persuasive tool to encourage people to join us in our mission to better inform the public. With this goal in mind, a copy of *Healthy Stories* has been donated to every accredited school of Public Health in Canada, Mexico and the United States.

Our stories have traveled across the nation as an educational tool, from Jacksonville, Florida to Los Angeles, California, in all levels of academia, from elementary schools to colleges and universities. Our story book has journeyed to members of the US Armed Forces stationed in Iraq, and Peace Corps volunteers in Ghana.

This year *Healthy Stories* focused on: chronic disease, nutrition, hurricane preparedness, sexually transmitted diseases, tuberculosis, HIV/ AIDS, domestic violence, environmental health, health promotion and fitness, WIC, women's health and community injury prevention and control.

We expanded into the area of public health poetry and nutritional recipes. *Healthy Stories* also continues to provide a bonus section in Creole and Spanish to our diverse community.

Hoping you find this year's compilation as fascinating, compelling and powerful as I did.

Lillian Rivera,
R.N., M.S.N., Ph.D.

Introduction

The editors take great pride in the publication of the third edition of *Healthy Stories* (HS). This year, we won a NACCHO model practice award, published our first newsletters, and graduated our first class of writers from Health Stories University. Our school of thought now has seven members. We have expanded our book's scope to include healthy poetry and recipe collections. In this edition, we have a number of firsts: a safety, a dental, a biographical, a hurricane and a spiritual story.

Marketing

Healthy Stories continues building its international marketing platform on the web. When you Google *"Healthy Stories."* we place in the first, second and fourth positions. Our stories have been picked up and published by others. We have sold numerous copies on Amazon.com, the Miami International Book Fair and the United States Conference on AIDS. Our books are also available for purchase through: BarnesandNoble.com, on eBay, Stylefeeder the Personal Shopping Engine, AbeBooks.com, Goodreads, ChainReading, Wikipedia under "Health Department", TheMedicineProgram, thedonald.net, Biblio, Alibris, TextbooksRus, Target and BookRenter.

Our readership can locate us at our websites: healthystories.net, healthystories.org or at the Miami-Dade Health Department's site, dadehealth.org under *Healthy Stories*.

A health care site in Edmonton, Canada has linked HS to their homepage.

Through our marketing efforts, our stories have become an invaluable tool to the field of public health.

Publicity

We have received favorable articles in:

The APHA, The Nation's Health
The NACCHO Exchange, Volume 7, Issue 4, fall 2008
The Florida Public Health Association, Fall issue 2008 newsletter; Volume 1 Issue 3
The South Florida Hospital News, October 2008

Southern University Chancellor's Report, Baton Rouge, Louisiana
El Nuevo Herald and *Miami Herald, Business Notes,* February 15, 2009
Miami-Dade County Health Department's Health Beat
Florida Department of Health—Health Advisor, March/April 2009

Community Service

We lectured to the North Miami Chamber of Commerce on the benefits to business of storytelling and to the 17th Annual University of Miami, Florida Bioethics Network Spring 2009 Conference, sponsored by the Miller School of Medicine, on the Role of Literature in Relation to Public Health and Ethics, "Why *Healthy Stories* Promote Good Health and Values."

We made the community healthier and happier by giving *Healthy Stories* copies as gifts or rewards to: retirees, employees of the month, new employees, hospital and nursing home patients, eagle scouts, soldiers, judges, police officers, school teachers, Peace Corp volunteers, medical students, visiting dignitaries from Detroit and Ann Harbor to San Francisco. Our book can be found in libraries as far away as Plymouth, New Hampshire.

In the spirit of friendship and cooperation we have given copies to our disaster preparedness partners in the CDC Quarantine Station and to Jackson Health System.

Education

A copy of *Healthy Stories* has been furnished to every accredited school of public health in the United States, Canada and Mexico.

All of the nation's public health associations received a holiday gift copy of our publication.

We have heard from Jacksonville's Baptist Health Infection Control and Employee Health nurses that they are sharing our hand washing poem with school children. The poem is also taught to kindergarten students in Los Angeles Unified School District.

To improve literacy, *Healthy Stories* can be found in the Florida Department of Health's "Read for Health" website.

Professors at Florida International University and the University of North Florida advise us that they continue to use our stories to inspire their public health students.

Wondrous Occurrences

Finding *Healthy Stories* published on an online Saudi Arabian encyclopedia medical site, www. SMSO.net.

Finding *Healthy Stories* being sold for British pounds on Langton Info Services, England.

Hearing a Palatka, Florida reader was so impressed with the book he cleared a shelf on his bookcase and dedicating the space solely to his copy of *Healthy Stories*.

Observing guests at the Florida Public Health Associate Conference lounging at their Orlando hotel pool reading their copy of *Healthy Stories* for hours.

Seeing *Healthy Stories* elevated to the status of coffee table book and also finding it in friends' bathrooms.

Meeting a participant at the NACCHO conference in Sacramento who when seeing our book exclaimed, "A year ago, I read those absorbing stories online at the CDC website."

Achieving the highest form of flattery, when we learned that two universities are contemplating publishing their own version of *Healthy Stories*.

Enjoying that one of our authors, Gerri LeClerc, received the Amazon Breakthrough Novel Award.

Rekindling the passion of writing for a twenty-year veteran of the North Miami Police force, upon hearing the history of *Healthy Stories*.

Granting permission for using our stories in sermons to a minister who was moved by our tales.

Seeing the following magical words appear on our Blackberries, "Greetings from Amazon.com Advantage You have a new order awaiting your confirmation."

One of our readers recommended to one of our writers, "Maybe you should quit your day job and become a full time writer."

Well, we are not quite ready to give up our day jobs at the Health Department, but we want to thank our loyal readers for their support and encouragement — and anyway, if we left the health department, where would our stories come from?

The Editors

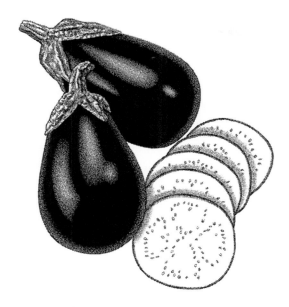

Armchair Eggplant

By Mort Laitner

I just learned I have been infected with a new disease.

I'm sitting in front of my computer typing a story when public health nurse walks in and instantly diagnoses my horrifying malady.

He glares down at me and says, "Be careful, you're developing a serious case of sitting disease."

I inquire, "What the heck is sitting disease?"

The nurse responds in a tone meant only for children, "Desk bounders, like you, only walk 5,000 steps a day. Outdoor working folk average 15,000 steps a day."

"You mean that I'm taking 10,000 less steps then those sanitarians out in the field?"

"Yup" he replies in a tone that acknowledges my higher math skills.

"Where are you getting all this scientific knowledge from?" I ask.

"Some Doc at the Mayo Clinic in Rochester. He says you need to do more walking, standing and moving around while you're working."

Now the nurse tests me like he imagines I have a rare case of "thinking disease."

"You must immediately increase your non-exercise activity thermogenesis."

"Say what?," I incredulously respond.

"You need to account for your daily movements and increase your caloric expenditures."

"You're not pulling my leg?"

"Nope, you heard of couch potatoes, haven't you?

"Yup."

"Well you're an armchair eggplant!"

"Has this Mayo doctor come up with any cures for sitting disease?" I wonder.

"Yup. Walk to lunch, have walk-and-talk meetings, pace while on the phone, stand when you talk to people, take the stairs. You can burn more calories each day. Make up for that 10,000 per day step deficiency. Just remember: YOU NEED TO MOVE MORE THOUGHOUT THE DAY."

I lift my body off the chair, stand up, then I walk up to this nurse while extending my hand. We shake and I say, "Thanks buddy, this sounds like it's going to be one fun activity. Let's walk to lunch. I have a sudden urge for baba ganoush."

Thanks to Heather VanNest, Tampa Bays10 for her story, Do you have "Sitting Disease?" and Dr. James Levine for his caring book, Move a Little, Lose a Lot.

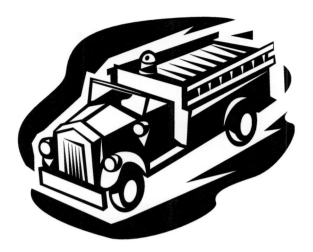

Safety Dance

By Bobby Glass

One bright and breezy Miami morning, I'm driving through an unfamiliar residential neighborhood. My windows are down, and I smell the sweet scent of freshly cut grass. Totally 80's Weekend on 97.3 FM blares tunes from the past on my radio. I laugh as I listen to a song titled "Safety Dance" by Men Without Hats. I haven't heard this song for years, and as a health department safety officer, I find the lyrics ironically titillating. I sing along.

Safety dance,
Safety dance,
Safety dance.

I drive past manicured yards with coconut palm tree fronds swaying and think how peaceful the neighborhood seems. In a fraction of a second, something catches my eye. I see a yellow Tonka toy truck and a relatively small object that looks like a toddler behind the tires of an SUV parked in a driveway. I glance at the house. The front door is open, but the screen door is closed. I think to myself and say "No it can't be". My mind reflects back to a three week-old news report about a child that was backed over and crushed to death by his mom's Hummer. My car is still rolling, and I think should I stop? What if I don't stop? Would I hear about the same account on the news? If I don't stop, would I be an accessory? What type of parent would enough to allow their child to play unsupervised behind this automobile? What if this was my child- would I want someone to stop?

I move my right foot from the gas to the brake pedal applying enough pressure to come to an abrupt stop and shift into park. Leaving my Prius, I slowly walk toward the driveway staring at the little boy in his pajama top and a diaper playing with his toy. I wonder now if the person responsible will have a confrontational attitude or be grateful. As I keep an eye on the youngster, I become angry thinking of all the things that could happen. I say hello to the toddler, and he just stares at me. I approach the front door and press down hard on the door bell. Taking out my frustrations, I ring it incessantly.

Ding dong,
Ding dong,
Ding dong.

As the silhouette of a mid-30's man dressed only in boxers approaches the door, I introduce myself, "Hi. My name is Bobby Glass and I work for the Miami-Dade County Health Department." I hand him my card that I just fished out of my wallet.

He replies with an aggravated tone, "Why are you ringing my bell so much? It's so early in the morning! I'm not interested in anything you're selling."

I politely respond, "No sir. I oversee the health department's safety program. Do you know that there is a small child playing underneath the Chevy SUV in your driveway?"

He shouts "NO!" and hurriedly makes his way out the screen door almost knocking me down. To this father's dismay, it was his eighteen-month old son still in pajamas who was last seen sleeping in his room; however, the boy snuck out.

As the child's mom comes out screaming and grabbing the child into her arms, tears of relief cascade down her cheeks.

The grateful father bear-hugged me and said, "I will never be able to thank you enough for saving my son's life."

I bite my tongue wanting to say, "I hope you learned your lesson", but quietly utter, "You're welcome," and walk away.

Getting back into my hybrid, I slowly push the ignition button and remember how I pressed the doorbell. With my hands on the steering wheel, I am elated for having done the right thing, being a good samaritan and possibly saving a life. I start singing again.

Safety dance,
Safety dance,
Safety dance.

Bobby Glass, MS, OHST is the Safety Program Manager for the Miami-Dade County Health Department.

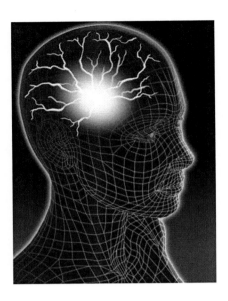

Ouch! Bet That Hurt!

By Phil Reichert

It was late 1979, when I was hired to be a "VD Investigator." That's how they referred to us at the time. It was venereal disease, and not sexually transmitted. Later we would be called, "STD Investigators," and eventually "DIS," or "Disease Intervention Specialists." Leave it to the government to come up with a title that would lead the general public to have no idea what you do for a living. Well, given the nature of the work, maybe that was a good thing.

We VDIs worked in the clinics every afternoon where we saw a variety of interesting and sometimes bizarre people who had a variety of interesting and sometimes bizarre problems with their plumbing. Mornings were spent driving around our appointed area searching out contacts to people who had syphilis and gonorrhea.

Even before the world had heard of Lorena Bobbit, there was a story in a local newspaper in the early eighties that reported on how a man had performed self-castration, then subsequently come to the realization that it was a bad idea and gotten himself to a hospital. He was triaged past the broken arms, minor knife and gunshot wounds and whisked into surgery where it was quickly and appropriately reattached. It was a good thing he remembered to bring it with him to the emergency room. According to the article, when asked why he had made the unusual amputation, he replied that voices had instructed him to chop it off because keeping it would just get him in trouble.

For months after the incident, during well-deserved breaks or lunches, someone in our group would still beg the question, "Why would someone do that?" Then the males around the table would cross our legs and in unison say, "Ouch!"

One day in clinic, I had just finished explaining to a patient how not to get re-infected. I would further explain the virtues of using a condom, especially if they were having sex with someone they just met. Depending on the disease we were addressing, the VDI might do an interview with the patient asking how to confidentially get in touch with their recent sexual partners so we could test and treat them. After repeating this information for the seventh or eighth time that day, one of the clinic nurses brought me the patient chart on a young man she had just treated. She asked me if I remembered the story from a year ago, about a fellow who had cut off his manhood and had it reattached. I replied, "Of course, didn't that subject just come up again during a coffee break last week?"

The nurse said, "I just treated him. You get to talk to him about prevention."

I exclaimed, "You treated him for what? Does it appear to work in the, well, normal way that it should?"

With a slight smile she replied, "Gonorrhea and Yes."

A man in his early to mid-twenties, that any woman and some men would find attractive, came into my office and I asked him to have a seat. I perused his medical record. The nurse had noted that she had taken a sample of the discharge that oozed from his privates. The lab tech had taken a look under the microscope and confirmed the gentleman was indeed infected with gonorrhea, a disease one obtains through sexual contact with an infected person. She had also noted as a sidebar, "Penis amputated and reattached approximately one year ago."

I asked the gentleman how he was doing and explained the virtues of abstinence or only having sex with only one non-infected partner, sometimes called mutual monogamy. If those were not options for him, I told him how valuable it might be to carry condoms with him at all times and use them correctly. He seemed well-educated, probably at least some college, and spoke intelligently. He seemed open to questions, at least a little bit, about the incident from the prior year.

I inquired, "Does everything work the way it did, uh, before the incident?"

"Yeah, I can pee and do everything I did before, but it's a little less responsive than it used to be."

"Just out of curiosity, and I'm sure you've heard this before, why did you do it?"

"Voices told me to do it. They said that having it would do nothing but cause me trouble, that I didn't really need it."

I thought to myself as he was leaving with a handful of condoms, Yep! A positive gonorrhea test, looks like it did get him in trouble. His voices were right and so were mine, "OUCH! I bet that hurt!"

Phil Reichert is currently the Program Administrator for the Hepatitis Prevention Program at the Division of Disease Control in Tallahassee.

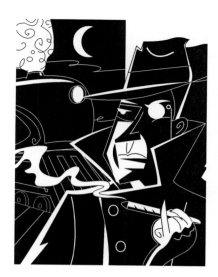

The Con Man[1]

By Morton Laitner

My friend Paul lies uncovered in his hospital bed, wrapped in a disposable diaper. His eyelids lazily droop, and I question if he is asleep.

"Paul," I choke back my fears as he does not respond, "Buddy, can you hear me?"

Deafening silence fills the room. I take my time to closely examine his bloated face, and then my eyes slowly take in his withered legs.

Touching his hand I repeat, "Paulie, can you hear me?"

He slowly opens his eyes. He gives me the look of ---now is my chance to tell him.

His words are garbled as oxygen is forced into his nostrils and a clear plastic mask rests on his face. In a staccato manner, he spits out his message.

"I was innocent...
You should have believed me...

---

1 The first known usage of the term "confidence man" was in 1849; it was used by the press during the trial of William Thompson. Thompson chatted with strangers until he asked if they had the confidence to lend him their watches, whereupon he would walk off with the watch; he was captured when a victim recognized him on the street. http://en.wikipedia.org/wiki/Confidence_trick

The cops never should have jailed me...
It was oxygen deprivation. Not dope!"

Paul now rests his eyes shut. He delivered his message.

Thirty days earlier, Paul had two strokes in rapid succession. Now his arms and one of his legs are paralyzed.

I think how ironic, throughout his life my old friend had two paralytic strikes against him.

Paulie was a con man with a dark karmic cloud which clung to him as if he was magnetized metal, constantly pointing his moral compass in the wrong direction.

He loved the confidence game. He exploited his friends, family, and acquaintances through their weaknesses and virtues.

I met Paul on the first day of law school. He was obnoxiously loud for his short stature – a younger white hybrid version of that eighties TV favorite George Jefferson and TV's favorite loser of the nineties George Costanza. He smoked incessantly as if his nervous system needed tobacco to thrive. Paul was a funny character, something right out of a Marvel comic book. Many of his classmates laughed with him, most at him. Paul desperately sought attention: a blend of insecurity, neurosis and dishonesty. He was a twin, and I rationalized his inordinate need for attention occurred when he and his brother shot out of the birth canal. Paul always acted like he would do anything for you. He not only acted, he did favors for people, but in his attempt to help he inexplicably made things worse. His heart seemed as big as his mouth. I never questioned his motives. I was the perfect mark.

Within a month he bragged, "I got hold of a telephone calling card. I'm charging calls all over the county for free."

I warned him, "You're going to get popped. All the phone company has to do is call your friends and ask who called you from New Orleans on such and such date." He laughed at my innocence. At first, he lied when busted by the phone company claiming it wasn't him. Later, he admitted his guilt and paid for a small portion of the calls.

A year later, he bragged, "Remember that Constitutional Law test that I said I got an 'A' on?"

"Yup, I could not believe you got a higher grade than me. I studied twice as hard as you did," I replied.

"Well, one of my friends gave me the test questions before the exam." He proudly recalled, "When I was called into the Dean's office for questioning, I claimed I never saw the questions."

Curiously I asked, "Did they make you take the test over?

His smile contorted into a smirk as he admitted, "I had to. I should have failed, but I ended up with a "C" in Con Law."

Paul was smart enough to get his law degree and pass a state bar exam. He married his college sweetheart and had a son. For the next ten years he made a living practicing criminal law.

Paul telephoned once or twice a year. "What's up bro? I bet you don't recognize my voice." He always bragged about his financial success. "I'm making money hand-over-fist. Life is real good. I got cases that are taking me all over the world." I knew from our law school days to cut whatever number he gave me in half to get a little closer to the truth. We laughed and reminisced about the good ol' days.

Then, two of Paul's old friends resurfaced: alcohol and drugs. They seeped into his soul. His old friends made him stop working. He tricked his clients into paying fees while neglecting their cases, as well as their telephone calls. For this negligent behavior, the state bar suspended his license. While under suspension he tried to con a police officer into not giving him a speeding ticket by pretending to be a practicing lawyer. It didn't work. He got the speeding ticket and lost his ticket to practice. Paul really did not lose it, he just flushed it away.

Now with no means of making an honest living, as well as his two destructive habits, Paul's hard-working wife wised up to his con game and gave up on him. She no longer would be his mark. She had lost confidence. She hoped and prayed he'd find a way to pay child support. He managed to make a few payments over the years. He even scammed himself into believing that his daily calls to his son made up for failing to support him.

Having represented the criminal element, Paul's next target was a big-time L.A. drug dealer. Paul became his jester, his defrocked mouth piece, his gopher and mule. In exchange for rendering these services, he earned his room, board and some pocket change to feed his habits.

One day, a shipment arrived at LAX. Paul's boss barked out an order. "Boy, here's the claim ticket, go to the airport, pick up the coke. It's in a red leather suitcase. You better not mess this up!"

Paul's hands shook as he reached out to take the stub and the car keys.

"Boss, I am east coast, can't one of the other guys do this? They know the airport better than I do."

The Boss laughed-out-loud, "Boy, it's time you earned your keep. Remember don't screw it up. There is hundred thousand dollars worth of dope in that suitcase. Every ounce of that dope better make its way into my grubby little hands. Do you hear me?"

Paul refused to look the boss in the eyes, staring at the tile floor as he whispered, "Yes, sir."

As Paul drove the Dodge, his nostrils flared smelling a rotten deal. He knew the odds were against him making it out of the airport without getting busted. The confidence man had no confidence. He was going to be the patsy. Feeling like a trapped rat, he knew his options were limited. Say no and die, or go to the airport and hope for the best. When Paul picked up the red leather suitcase, he walked ten paces before he heard, "Put the suitcase down and slowly put your arms in the air." Paul complied. He begged, "I was just doing a favor for a friend. I don't know what's in the bag!" In front of his eyes, the suitcase was opened exposing two cellophane wrapped bricks of cocaine hidden in some old shirts.

The lead cop yelled, "There's enough coke here to get you twenty years in the slammer. You'll die in jail, punk." The officer looked at one of the rookie cops and demurely said, "Throw this clown in a cell and I'll talk to him in a few hours."

Paul thought about demanding a lawyer and then thought better of it. He was led away in handcuffs as tears streamed down his cheeks. The small-time con artist was going to do big time.

True to his word, the officer showed up in Paul's cell four hours after his arrival. Paul's face bloated from crying. His eyes were as red as the leather suitcase. The cop held Paul's history in his hands, "You're a pathetic loser, a con man without a brain. You've lost your career, your wife, your kid and now your freedom," pausing to slowly enunciate, "for a long time."

Paul knew what was going to be the next words out of the police officer's mouth. "You rat on your buddies right now or we're going to ask the DA to charge you with felony possession with intent to distribute. You will be lucky to be out in the year 2012." He looked into Paul's puffy eyes knowing he had flipped him as easily as a McDonald's burger.

Paul did not stop squealing for the next two hours as the stenographer took down every word. He chain smoked only stopping for coughing attacks which slowed the flow of his confession. He begged the officer, "I need a drink; my throat is parched." Only to be told, "Con man, there is water on the table. That's all you're getting."

Paul had cut the deal of his life. In exchange for his testimony against the boss and his gang, Paul would not go to jail. He would be put in a witness protection program and given a new name and identity.

Paul knew that if boss' people found him before the trial, it would be the last deal of his life. When the boss was sentenced to twenty years, Paul was driving a cab in Atlanta.

The con man could not leave well enough alone. He started to gripe that the feds were not providing him with all they promised. He threatened to sue. And when he finally filed a claim against the Federal Government, he was thrown out of the program.

Paul realized his scamming skills could be put to the test as a used car salesman. He was right for a while; however, when the local economy headed south, so did Paul.

When Paul came to visit me, he asked, "How about a loan? I promise to pay you back."

I laughed a little too loudly, "Do I look like a subprime banker? If I gave you money it would ruin our friendship. You would never pay me back."

He replied, "How about getting me a job at the health department?"

"Paul, I don't think the health department has any jobs for a person with your skill set or qualifications. You are over qualified. Talk to me after you get a license."

How do you tell a con man/friend he is not welcome at your place of employment?

How do you tell a con man/friend that just because he lives on the internet, he's not qualified to teach abstinence or safe-sex?

How do you convince yourself that maybe this loser should not be your friend? Aren't we all given a cross to bear?

Paul was always invited over for holiday meals. He brought his contagious laugh, his uncontrollable cough, and his signature dish of baked beans.

A few years later, Paul's Florida used car salesman career ended in failure. He was getting evicted; his car repossessed, and was losing his girlfriend, Mary, a washed-out sullen-faced recovering alcoholic. They met at an AA meeting. Mary had seen the dark side of life and was crawling toward the light. Mary put up with Paul's shenanigans for a few months, but dumped him when she realized he was scamming her out of her hard-earned cash. Paul could not and would not let go. He phoned her twelve times a day begging, "Please let me see you, just one more time. I'll do anything for you. I love you!"

Her response was clear, "It's over! Stop calling me. Stop harassing me. If you don't stop, I'm calling the cops. I'll have you arrested!" Mary yelled, "I don't love you!" as she slammed down the receiver.

Paul's family had given up on him years earlier. Not even his son could or would rescue him. Paul's last resort was me. The phone rang, "Buddy, how about letting me stay on your couch until I work things out?"

I sadly responded, "Paul, sorry there is no room for you in my home. The last time you stayed in my home, I literally had to throw you and your stuff out the door. Don't tell me you forgot."

"Well, since I don't have any wheels, how about a ride to the homeless shelter?" he replied.

I answered, "I'll pick you up at your apartment in one hour. Be ready to leave when I get there."

When I approached the apartment, I noticed the yellow sheriff's three day eviction notice taped on the door. I walked into the studio which looked and smelled like a saloon. The room had not been cleaned in over a year. Empty beer cans and full ashtrays littered the floor. I wondered what it would have taken to get Paul to throw this mess into the dumpster. Sarcastically I said, "You sure know how to leave an apartment."

Of course he had not packed his bags. I touched his desktop

computer feeling the heat of use. As I waited, I pondered, "Does he think I am such a sucker that I'll drive him to my house?" My angry silence did not bode well for his last hope.

Wordlessly, we drove toward the shelter. He shattered our silence with stoic words, "I'm going to treat this trip as another of life's adventures. I'm a survivor. I should write my autobiography. It would sell a million copies and be on the New York Times best seller list."

I smiled thinking, Paul, writing a book requires work; a word which shies away from your very being. Who will you trick into authoring it?

Seeing a diner on the side of the road, I pulled over and offered him a last supper. He ate his steak sandwich as if he was a condemned man. He washed it down with merlot. He belched out a loud, "Thanks for the meal buddy."

At the locked gates of the homeless shelter, I gave Paul a big bear hug and bid him farewell, "Good luck! Try to be good!"

He signed in, looked straight ahead and with valise in hand marched past the now opened gate. He yelled back, "Don't forget to call."

Later, I heard from him that the shelter wanted to kick him out for violations of house rules. Paul was wheeling and dealing cigarettes and favors with the residents. His catch-me-if-you-can attitude was not appreciated by the staff. Before they threw him out, Paul collapsed.

His years of smoking lead to emphysema. His lungs were shot and now infected. Unable to breathe, he was knocking on death's door. His son visited him and found hit hard to express his love, even though Paul was near death, hooked up to tubes pumping oxygen into his collapsed lungs. With my coaxing, Paul's son touched his hand beseeching him to get well. Someone was listening.

A miraculous recovery opened the door of his next scam. He applied for Social Security disability and got it. The government check paid his rent and minimal provisions. He acted like he had just won the lottery. No more homeless shelters for him. He scammed a doctor with his back pain story to obtain governmentally funded narcotics. He grew old and obese on the government's dime. His meager dole put him on a high-carb diet. He gained thirty pounds, only exercising his fingers on the keyboard or pressing down on his mouse while playing video games or searching for love online. To my amazement, women online had con-dar (radar against con men) that protected them from this ilk. One exception was a stylish fifty-year old deceiver who managed to trick him into driving to North Miami Beach for dates. He spent his last three hundred dollars dating her. She suckered him with the promise of love. The con man never even got a kiss.

He was more successful with Sally, an elderly black woman, who lived in his apartment complex. In exchange for driving her to doctor's appointments, he was allowed to drive her car whenever he needed it. When he smacked into a telephone pole with damages to the tune of $500, Paul said to Sally, "I'll repair it sweetheart." When Sally demanded, "Paul, when are you going to fix my car?" For months he replied, "Soon Sally, my dear." He never did repair the vehicle. He simply ignored her requests until she gave up.

Thirty days before Paul's my visit to the hospital, my phone rang at 8:30 on Sunday morning. An unfamiliar feminine voice said, "Hi, I'm Jane, a neighbor of Paul's and he's locked up." She continued, "He was charged with DUI. The police tested him while he was hospitalized and found drugs in his blood. The idiot drove his car into another telephone pole. Now, they moved him to the jail. He asked me to call you to bail him out."

I inquired, "What's the bail?"

"Five thousand dollars," Jane replied. "All you need to come up with is five hundred to a bail bondsman."

"Jane, give me your phone number please." I scribbled down her number and told her I'd call her back after I thought it over.

What would Moses, Jesus, or Mohammad do? Am I my brother's keeper? I opined that all three would say bail your friend out. What about Dr. Phil? Tough love. I called my friend, Lawrence, who practices criminal law. He speculated that Paul would be released by the judge within two days. He continued, "But it isn't a large sum of money and why not just bail him out?"

My wife and I discussed the pros and cons over freshly brewed coffee, and finally, she said, "Paul will not even show up for the bond hearing, and we will be out $5,000 bucks." As I balanced all of these thoughts, I contemplated out loud Sally's automobile predicament,

"Paul has no respect for other people's money or property." We nodded our heads in agreement, and I remarked as I sipped my coffee, "Paul will trick the guards to put him into the hospital. He's got emphysema. And besides, he'll be out in two days."

I phoned Jane, "Sorry, I've decided not to help Paul."

I had decided that our friendship had to come to an end. I never thought I'd see Paul again.

Now as I'm walking out of the hospital, I formulate my response to his guilt-trip message.

I was innocent.

Paul, your innocence is not the issue; the issue is your lack of character.

You should have believed me.

How could I believe you when your whole life has been a lie?

The cops never should have jailed me.

Maybe the police shouldn't have arrested you, but there were drugs in your blood – sounds like probable cause.

It was oxygen deprivation. Not dope!

Paul, it may have been oxygen deprivation. But, I'm sorry; your old friend no is longer a dope.

As I lie in my comfortable bed, wrapped in a quilt of memories, my eyelids lazily droop and I ponder how Paul is doing...

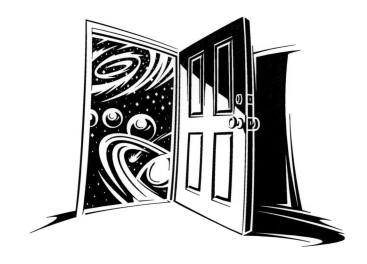

People are Strange

By John Holmes

I hate Monday mornings. Arriving at the office at 7:30 AM to unlock the door and disarm the security system, my routine is so predictable. On comes the computer to check today's schedule and any email I missed on my Blackberry. I read my Microsoft outlook calendar - November 27. I focus in on the number. I recall Morrison, Joplin and Hendrix all died in their 27th year. The trinity all had abused substances. I think how addicted I am to coffee. I wish somebody would be here before me to make a pot. I will make a note to tell my office assistant she needs to have my coffee ready when I arrive (just kidding). I just want my java! I hear the staff arriving one by one. They are grateful that "someone" has already started the brew. The stories of their weekend adventures have already started. It is always pretty much the same: Spouse problems, bad dates, somebody had a party, or it was just another boring weekend.

The first phone call and it is not 8:00 AM yet. I wait to see how many rings before the phone is answered. Only three rings, somebody must be in a good mood. The call is a complaint (surprise) about a bag of used hypodermic needles dumped along the road. I think this is a strange human behavior to litter our highways with agents of death. Ironic my earlier thoughts about the dead rock idols and now a call about needles. After talking to my lead inspector, we decide to go to the site together to see if we can just pickup the sack and that will be that. I am always concerned when it comes to needles because a "stick" can happen so easily. My lead inspector changes his mind about being my copilot so I depart alone to clean up the mess before anything happens.

As I am driving the county truck to where I think the syringes were dumped, my mind starts to wander when my radio starts to play "Riders on the Storm". I am instantly spiraled back to 1969.

I was waiting for a bus to downtown San Francisco. My transistor radio played top 40 tunes, what we now call "Golden Oldies". A news story came on about how they are trying to stop the spread of disease with a needle exchange program. They would start a trial program in Haight-Ashbury. I remember thinking that was a strange way to stop the spread of disease. Why not just get the hippies off hard drugs? My favorite song "Light My Fire" by The Doors burned into my ears. The announcer interrupted the song to remind the audience that The Doors were performing that night in San Francisco's Winterland Ice Rink. I could not believe my luck that The Doors were performing on my night off. I decided to go see my favorite group led by my favorite singer, Jim Morrison.

That night, I walked up and down the steep hill streets, taking in the feel of the city that night for a few hours until it was time to get in line to see Jim. I was excited just to be there. Time passed and the line shortened. I was finally inside. On the main floor, I picked a spot to stand where I could see well and not so close that I had to look up all night.

This would be one of the greatest nights of my life. I stood within 25 feet of Jim Morrison. The mood of the arena changed as The Doors were about to perform. A pot-haze cloud formed a couple feet above the floor which unlocked my doors of perception.

It got really quiet as the The Doors sauntered onstage. They started to play a song, but no Jim! I hoped he was not in jail again. He had just been arrested earlier that week at Miami's Dinner Key Auditorium. Then I saw him. The Lizard King wore his signature leather pants and black shirt. His unbuttoned ruffled shirt exposed his chest. The band shifted to play "Touch Me", followed by "Love Her Madly." The crowd screamed in excitement, and I was even more electrified because Jim was drinking a Bud. I could not believe Morrison and I drank the same beer. Jim was drinking Bud and singing at the same time. Here was the greatest performer I had ever seen. As I tried to get his attention, my shouts were drowned out by the crowd. I shouted, "Share your Bud." Not realizing that the song was over, I just kept yelling. Mr. Mojo Risin' heard my pleas. In true Morrison fashion, he threw the can of beer at me. It hit me right in the middle of my chest. Momentarily dazed, I somehow managed to pick up the can of beer. I then did what any Morrison fan would do. I guzzled it down. I shared a Bud with Jim Morrison.

My mind has wandered so far that I miss my turn to where the needles have been dumped. I turn the truck around and try to find the location. Pulling off the road I check the map, and the page I need had gotten wet and is unreadable. I spy an attractive woman waiting for a bus. As I ask her for directions, my mind again wanders; this time to Paris in 2007.

As I watched the women walk by on the sidewalk of the Champs Elysées, I asked my wife, "Where are we going next?

She replied, "We're headed to the Arc De Triomphe and the Eiffel Tower. If we have time, we'll see Moulin Rouge, the Louvre, and the Basilique Du Sacre-Coeur. We have a full schedule today."

However, the place I had to see before we left Paris was the "Cimetiere Pere Lachaise", the city's most famous cemetery.

As I climb back into the county truck, I thank the attractive woman for the directions. My mind is not on work, but I have to get back to the investigation. I finally arrive where the needles were dumped. As luck would have it, most of the needles are still in a container, and the few that are on the ground, I am able to pick up without being pricked.

But my mind is still stuck in Paris. My wife and I were tired of touring, but I was determined to go to "Cimetiere Pere Lachaise." I told my wife, "My interest in this cemetery is because Jim Morrison is buried there, and I need to see his grave. I have some unfinished business with him."

My wife replied, "We can make the stop but it will have to be quick." I nodded my head in agreement.

I detoured into a market claiming a deep thirst to my wife and hid a beer in my coat pocket. When we arrived at the cemetery, I found, in a corner of the cemetery, a simple grave site - only a headstone. I was glad that we were the only people there as we stood at his grave. I popped the lid on the beer, took a large swig and slowly poured the rest on the grave. As I murmured, "Jim, thanks for the poetry, the music and the memories. I hope you enjoy this French beer as much as I enjoyed your Bud."

As the golden liquid puddled on the hallowed ground, the dry earth drank in the intoxicant. The acrid odor rose hitting our nostrils. My wife gazed into my eyes and with a wry smile said, "Morrison was right, people are strange. Then she wrapped her arms around me and whispered in my ear, "Je t'aime."

John Holmes is the Environmental Health Director in Putnam County Florida, and he was the Healthy Stories 2008 Best Story Competion winner.

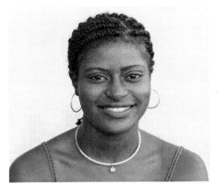

Undetectable

By Sonjia Kenya

Deidre lives in the hood. She waves from the top of her steep metal stairway and yells, "Come on up." Wearing a dirty t-shirt with uncombed hair and an infectious smile, Deidre invites me in. I follow her into the living room, examining the tiny dark apartment. I hope I am doing this discreetly, trying to look at things closely while pretending not to look at all. A tiny, white barking mutt runs toward me. I see fleas jumping through his coat. I'm allergic to fleas, but oblige Deidre when she requests, while she runs into her bedroom, "Please pet my dog." Much to my already itchy eyes' dismay, the trip to the bedroom was to retrieve a mother cat nursing five kittens inside of a cardboard box. After introductions to the cat and each kitten, Deidre attempts to give me a kitten but I protest and refrain from scratching at the fleas I imagine are crawling through my mane of curly hair. Deidre exudes warmth that is hard not to reciprocate.

I am here because Deidre left the hospital with a viral load of less than 350 and a T-cell count of over 1000. My job is to reduce health disparities and enroll her into our HIV adherence study. I begin the interview,"When were you first diagnosed? She replies, "I was first diagnosed positive in 2004 but didn't believe it until 2006 when I got real sick and was in the emergency room." She continued, "I don't have any health benefits and I don't take my meds because they give me a rash. I get so sick, I frequently visit the emergency room and I'm often hospitalized." I ask about her personal history, and Deidre says, "I've been clean for two years. I had two kids but I haven't seen them for months. My boyfriend is responsible for taking care of me. Sometimes we have unprotected sex although he knows I'm infected. He claims to be HIV negative. He also claims he's not cheating on me but I'm not so sure." Deidre lives with him and another male who is her best friend that also likes her romantically. Neither is home right now.

Some days she does not leave the apartment because the stairs from the street are too much for her. Everyone in the building knows she's HIV positive. She asks me to feel her thighs because she believes the virus is changing her body and wants reassurance because she feels her thighs don't look quite right. I finish the interview and tell her I will assign a community health promoter to her case who will contact her shortly to begin helping her improve HIV adherence behaviors. She asks, "Can you assign one that is just like you?" I smile, and we hug. I walk down the steep metal stairs without holding the rail.

Three months later, Deidre moved to a new house. It is a one story, three-bedroom home where she lives rent-free in exchange for caring for the elderly owner. The neighborhood is better than her last, and I walk into the unlocked screen door without knocking to find a bright, well-furnished, spacious home. I hear her laughing and talking with Teikia, the health promoter I assigned to her case. Deidre immediately walks over and hugs me as I notice her hair neatly contained in a ponytail and her clean T-shirt tucked into fitted jeans that show off her curvy figure. Remembering how many antihistamines I had to take after our last visit, I ask about the animals. She has cut down to only one cat who beckons to her call when she opens the back door, exposing a manicured yard. The UPS delivery truck pulls up with a delivery box from the satellite TV company, and she handles receipts and delivery paperwork like a practiced professional. Deidre smiles like a kid on Christmas. As she opens the box, her cheeks come alive revealing her natural beauty, and I notice her white teeth sparkle against her rich, dark skin. I am here to ask her to make a public presentation to my board of directors, a group comprised of philanthropists, the dean of the medical school and medical professors. She exclaims, "Teikia has already told me about it, and I'm excited about sharing my story."

She shows me the outfit she's planning to wear, and her dangling earrings swirl as she describes how healthy she feels as a result of Teikia's help with medical adherence.

I complement her, "Your new home is a lot better than your last place."

She agrees, "Its better but I'm planning on getting my own place using my own paychecks."

She describes her new exercise routine and invites me to feel her thighs, which she says are back to normal. "I've reunited with my children two months ago. Why don't you have kids?" she asks. She tells me about her love and gratitude for Teikia's help getting health insurance, learning to make her own medical appointments, getting prescriptions and feeling important enough to want to take care of herself. I self-indulge and remind her that she asked for a health promoter just like me; Teikia lets me bask in her glory for just a second.

We begin preparing her speech for the board, and I learn that she wants to write a book to help other women like her overcome their illness. The title is "How I Got Over." We plan her speech to be concise and discuss strategies to curtail nervous jitters.

At the board meeting, I conclude my program update by introducing Teikia and Deidre to confirm our study progress. Teikia describes amazing changes Deidre has made and congratulates her success. Deidre shines bright in her silky, flowing pantsuit with perfect make-up, matching earrings and shoes. After a glorious smile, she admits that she's nervous and must refer to her notes.

I give Deidre an encouraging smile as she starts her speech, "I love these two beautiful young ladies. When I met Teikia and Sonjia, I didn't care about anything. I didn't care about life. I was gone. But now I'm living. I was unhappy and now I'm happy. I was unhealthy and now I'm healthy. I was underserved. Now I'm undetectable. And now I'm in the process of writing a book. It's called, "How I Got Over". I want to write it to educate other people like me. I want to share my story to let them know they can get better. They can be healthy too. And when I'm done with that," she pauses to look at her health promoter standing to the left, "You better watch out Teikia, cuz' I'm taking your job."

Sonjia Kenya, MA, MS, EdD is an assistant professor at University of Miami, School of Medicine, and a program manager for health dispanties research.

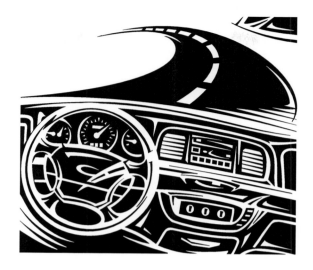

You Led a Good Life

By Mort Laitner

I t was one of those days where my life's real troubles were apt to be things that never crossed my worried mind; the kind of day where I was literally blindsided at 9 AM on an idle Tuesday morning.[1]

At 8 AM, I voted in the Bush-Clinton presidential election. At 8:30 AM, I cruised, top down, in my spanking-brand-new blue Miata. As the cool November breeze parted my hair, the sun baked the top of my head. I smiled the smile of a trouble-free man driving his mid-life toy. No need for the radio to be on, this picture needed no background music.

Damn it!

I heard the mood-breaking, troubling beeps emanating from my pants pocket. The digital number displayed on my beeper was a co-worker, followed by our emergency code. As I pulled off I-95, I worried about finding a pay-phone in this dangerous neighborhood. I found one and, of course, it was broken. The next phone I located worked, but my co-worker failed to pick up.

Machine: "This is the Department of Health and Rehabilitative Services, please clearly enunciate your name, phone number and message after the beep."

1 A modification of the song "Everybody's free (to wear sunscreen)" by Baz Luhrmann heard in the movie "The Big Kahuna"

As my mood shifted into negative mode, I responded in a firm tone, "If you beep someone with an emergency, please try to be near your phone so you can respond," slamming down the receiver in an act of frustration.

At 8:45 AM, fifteen minutes wasted, I jumped back in my car, clicking on my seat belt, as I started driving toward the 401 building. I remembered the promise I made to that state trooper three months earlier who was about to write me a ticket for failure to wear the belt. "Officer, as a fellow state employee, I promise you from this day on, I will always wear my seat belt when behind the wheel of my automobile."(The promise worked; I didn't get the ticket.)

At 8:58 AM, I felt the beeper in my shirt pocket. I screamed, "I HATE PEOPLE WHO YELL EMERGENCY WITHOUT WAITING FOR A RESPONSE!" (You can do this in a convertible on I-95 and no one but G-d hears you.)

At 8:59 AM, catharsis, the scream worked. I felt much better as I turn off the freeway. I was two blocks away from my office.

At 9:00 AM, I drove under the overpass. Shadows in dark shades of grey reflected on the cement pillars as I waited for the light to change. Green appeared. I inched forward as I glanced to my right. I saw a ten ton truck running the red light right into me. I enter a slow motion world. I heard a deafening screech of brakes. Then, the loudest crash I had ever heard.

I blacked out as my brain shifted into pause.

In total darkness, an inner voice said, "You're dead."

The voice then said the five most important words I ever heard, "You led a good life."

Now the viewing screen in my mind imagined a large VCR and a heavenly finger pushing down on the play button. The VCR and the hand disappeared, only to be replaced by black and white twirling clouds. These clouds formed a tornado. This speeding funnel disappeared as my eyes began to focus on the exploded air-bag. The smell of burning rubber and noxious gasses burned my nostrils as my body rattled from the blow of the air-bag.

I had to get out of the car.

I WAS ALIVE!

Next thought, am I a quadriplegic?

Moving my left hand pinkie finger on the door handle, I appreciated that I have control of one of my hands.

Next thought, am I a paraplegic?

Slowly I popped the lock and the Miata door opened. Breathing in toxic fumes, I said a silent prayer, "Please G-d let me get out of this car."

I scanned my body for injuries. As I looked for blood, I only saw a small scratch on my ring finger from which one tear-shaped droplet of blood flowed.

With all the energy I could muster, I pushed my body out of the wreck.

I screamed and jumped for joy, "I'm the luckiest man--- I'm alive--- I'm not paralyzed!"

Standing next to me was the lady whose car the truck slammed my car into. In amazement she asked, "Are you okay?"

"Am I okay? I am the luckiest person in Miami!," I bellowed.

She eye-balled my destroyed vehicle not appreciating my love of life and health.The police arrived and issued the truck driver a ticket.

Then the ambulance arrived. The paramedics examined me. As I lay on their stretcher with a blood pressure cup strapped to my arm, I studied my ring finger. I couldn't believe what I observed. Miraculously, the scratch and the blood had vanished. The paramedics recommended I go to the hospital for further tests. I declined their offer, still mystified over what happened to the cut.

As I walked the two remaining blocks to my office, I reflected on how the airbag and the seatbelt saved my life. I marveled at the sun's rays piercing though the clouds. I wondered out loud, "Had I really led a good life?" For the third time that day, I stared at my ring finger which triggered the memory of that heavenly finger pushing down on the VCR play button. On that cool November day, I no longer worried about my life's troubles because I knew the answer.

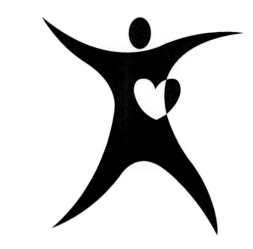

Helpless Heart

By Gerri LeClerc

I'll call her June because that is the month she died. We worked together in a small covert office for one of the intelligence communities. This type of work creates families as well as colleagues; we are under oath to keep government secrets and can only discuss our work with each other. As a result, we work tightly together and make deep relationships that often last a lifetime. June's lifetime was too short, too unhappy, and her work family was unable to prevent her death.

June spoke to me me because I was a nurse; though I was not working in a clinical position, she knew I would keep her confidence. Her problem had been diagnosed by our co-worker and psychologist, Doctor Mike. June was a deeply depressed battered woman. She'd been in her situation for years and at the time I became involved she was in a stage of psychological paralysis, helplessness.

I am not an expert in any way on battered woman syndrome, though it has always frustrated me, as a nurse and a woman, when a spouse cannot escape an abusive husband. Even as June's personal experience was opened to me, it only confused me more.

Women, in just one generation, have achieved stellar goals in our society. We recently had our first woman candidate for president.

We've made strides in equal pay, military combat, as CEOs, doctors, lawyers and business owners. These changes in a woman's freedom and financial independence have not significantly reduced our submission to abuse or the number of deaths related to it. Why?

June was well-educated and respected in our organization. She kept to herself; was pleasant, and we thought shy. When she talked to me about herself, it was as if she were discussing someone else. She imparted only small tidbits of her situation, and always rationalized her husband's behavior. She spoke of their mutual love for each other, which was her reason for not leaving him. She knew intellectually that her depression was caused by the abusive relationship, but she was unable to walk away.

Battered women often feel guilt or responsibility for their partner's anger. Even if she recognizes the beatings she receives are unjustified, she often stays to try to repair the marriage. June felt hopeless to resolve her own situation, instead she turned inside herself and became depressed. Perhaps her spouse had threatened suicide, or maybe he threatened to take away her children or told her he would kill her if she left. I don't know. We have all seen the sad numbers on abuse related deaths; we have all been affected by news stories of men who murdered their wives.

The last time I remember June with hope in her eyes and a smile on her face was her last Christmas. Our office had a crazy gift exchange called a Yankee Swap. Everyone brought a gift and got a number. Number one started and chose a gift, opened it. Number two opened a gift and had the choice of keeping it or taking number one's gift. And so it goes until the last person. There are always some returned treasures, a laminated pizza slice, an ugly lamp, or a ladies retro hat. The laughter never quits and that year, June joined in, laughing and enjoying the time with her work family.

As the snows melted, a breathtaking Virginal spring emerged. Flowering Bartlett Pears, Forsythia, Azaleas, and Rhododendron turn our area into a wonderland of color, but is also a damp and cloudy time. Overwhelming beauty can make a depressing contrast if your life is not happy. I think it may have for June.

As she moved deeper into her depression, Doctor Mike asked my assistance in convincing June to undergo electroshock therapy. He was very worried about her and thought the treatment might be effective for her. I did my part and June agreed to have the treatment. One month later, June took her own life.

I'm sharing a little of June's plight so that I may touch even one life in trouble. Unlike years ago, there are a myriad of organizations set up to help any victim of domestic violence. The internet is a source of knowledge of every aspect of assistance available to anyone who needs it. (If you're in an abusive situation, access information from a computer at the library or other safe place, not from your home.) Call the National Domestic Violence Hotline at 1-800-799-SAFE (7233) to find information or crisis centers near you. Please, there are people waiting to help you—don't settle for abuse; don't become a number! You deserve to fulfill your own life and no one in the world has the right to hurt you. ☼

Gerri LeClerc is an author, nurse and previously worked for the CIA.

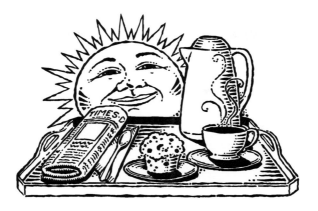

Steam Lining

By Mort Laitner

Eastern sunlight streams into the café. Hot beams of light flood the room. Beads of sweat trickle down my face. As I attempt to read my Writer's Digest, out of the corner of my vision, I observe dark quivering lines of steam shadows dancing on the white spaces of the magazine page. I pick up the coffee cup disturbing my darting dancers. The rich Arabica flavor leaves a slight bitterness on my tongue. I place the mug in the same spot on the table so the steam floats above black-ink brew and is struck by the rays. The shadows magically reappear. Crescent-moons bounce on and off the table.

The reflections, like shadows on a cave wall, cause me to ponder their meaning. People, like these shadows, make brief appearances: seconds, minutes, hours, a day in our lives. One of these shadowy people appeared thirty-three years ago in mine. He only appeared for one hour but I will never forget him.

In my first year of practice, I worked for the Legal Aid Society of Baton Rouge, Louisiana. One of my clients, a middle-aged white woman, wore clothes that reeked of tobacco. Her facial architecture displayed years of hard drinking, smoking and living. She curled her lips and exhaled smoke rings in my direction as if she was trying to lasso my nose.

"My ex-husband is a worthless lump of coal. All the bum does is drink all day long. I don't know the last time he held a job."

I asked, "Did you bring your divorce decree?"

She opened her purse, shuffled through the bag, and whipped out the final judgment. "Here it is," she said as she handed the papers to me.

"I see the judge awarded you ten dollars a week in alimony."

"Yup," she replied. "And he hasn't paid me in thirteen weeks. That son of a six shooter owes me a $130. The ten bucks a week allows me to buy two cartons of Marlboros. If he doesn't pay me, I want him jailed. I want him to stay there until he knows the names of every cockroach in his cell."

"Miss, I'll draw up the contempt of court motion, and we should be in court next week. We'll teach your ex a lesson he won't forget."

My client puckered her lips, blew another perfect circle in my direction; the smoke magically dissipated before my eyes. She gave me that look of "I can't wait to see what happens in court."

The week passed quickly. At 9:00 AM the bailiff called the case. My heart beat faster than a tom-tom drum. I had never jailed anyone before. I called the ex to the witness stand, and he was sworn in. He looked haggard, like a man who had been stepped on throughout his life. He carried the demeanor of a frightened man who would give anything for a drink. He was barely 50 going on 80.

Before I opened my mouth, a smile grew across my face. I made the realization that all my hard work and money to get a degree and a license had culminated in my efforts to imprison an alcoholic so that his ex-wife could purchase enough cigarettes to take her down the lung cancer highway.

After the preliminary questions I asked:

Lawyer: Sir, do you drink alcoholic beverages?

Defendant: Yes sir.

Lawyer: What type of alcoholic beverages do you drink?

Defendant: Beer.

Lawyer: How much beer do you consume on a daily basis?

Defendant (looking into judge's eyes): Your honor, in the morning I open a can of Budweiser. I drink half the can, and I put the rest back in the fridge. Later in the day, I finish that can of Bud.

I watched as the judge's face darkened. The judge, being a drinking man, didn't like this sworn witness' bold face lies.

Judge: Sir, I think I've heard enough. I think your testimony has been less than forthright. I'm going to order that you be jailed until you pay your ex-wife the $130 of alimony you owe her.

He hammered his gavel ending the case.

As the bailiff handcuffed the ex and walked him toward the jailhouse, I noticed tears glistening down his face. I felt terrible. A man was losing his freedom because of my actions. My client was jubilant and gave me a bear hug of gratitude.

Approximately five hours later, I received a call from the ex's brother. He told me he had the $130 and begged me to get his brother out of jail. I advised him to bring the cash to my office, and I would do my best to get his brother out that night. I succeeded in getting the judge to sign an order releasing the ex. By 7:00 PM he was out of jail, and my burden lifted like the smoke from my client's cigarettes.

I only heard from my client one more time. She called sobbing and said, "My man is dead. My ex, the day after he was released from the jail died of a heart attack."

My chest tightened with the knowledge that a man that I helped imprison died in less than 24 hours after his release.

As I sit in the café looking at the tiny reflections floating on pages of the magazine, I ponder how people come in and out of our lives for short periods of time but some leave indelible tattoos on our soul.

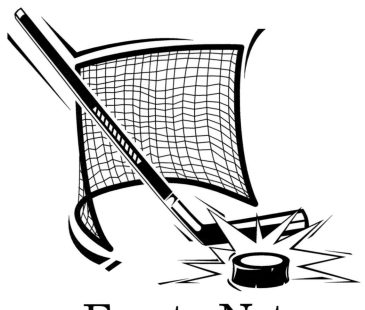

Empty Net

By Amy Tejirian

As he studied his face in the mirror of the locker room bathroom, he thought to himself, "I hope no one can notice. I need to do this. I have persevered through more pain. They are counting on me." His chest felt like a freight train had collided with it at 100 miles per hour. His thin, pale face did not show any signs of his hurting, his fatigue or the chills that ran through his 5'6", 185 pounds frame. He had earned the nickname, "Le Concombre de Chicoutimi" (The Chicoutimi Cucumber). Because of this thin stature and his composed character, he was as cool as a cucumber. He pulled on his famous blue, white and red toque and started to make his way to the ice.

"Go Habs Go! Go Habs Go!" (Habs is a nick name for the Montréal Canadiens, which is a shortened term for their nickname "Les Habitants".) The incessant chant grew louder and with more fervor as Georges Vézina approached the rink. The hometown crowd had been anxiously waiting all summer and fall for this day, the 1925-26 Montréal Canadiens season opener. When they spotted their beloved goalkeeper step onto the ice, the crowd exploded.

Georges calmly skated towards the net. Sweat rolled down his forehead and cheeks. He wiped it away with his sleeve. Some chest pain and a fever weren't going to stop him from enjoying his favorite activity. Georges had been the Canadiens goalie for the past 15 years and never missed a single game. Even when the Stanley Cup finals were canceled in 1919 due to the Spanish flu epidemic, Georges was prepared to stop any puck that flew his way. And Habs fans loved his passion and dedication. They recognized he was the greatest goalie hockey had ever seen. They celebrated the first shutout game that he had accomplished, the very first shutout in the NHL. How could Georges let them down today just because he wasn't feeling 100 percent? The rambunctious crowd made Georges forget about his ailments. He stood stoically in front of the net. Georges was ready – "Bring it on!"

The puck dropped. The Canadiens won the face-off against their opponents, the Pittsburgh Pirates. The Habs players skated away from Georges as they tried to score a goal, but to no avail. The puck rebounded off the goal post, and a Pirates player stole the puck. This large man in yellow and black broke away from the rest of the pack, puck in hand. He raced across the rink, past center ice and into the Habs zone. Quickly, only inches from the goal, he drew back his stick slightly and tried to shoot in the round, vulcanized rubber disc into the net. Instinctively, Georges deflected the puck, slightly moving his arm that clutched his stick. The spectators burst into a deafening cheer, "Go Habs Go! Go Habs Go!"

This non-stop action continued throughout the whole first period. Every time a Pirate tried to shoot a goal, Georges did not disappoint his fans. They praised his skill and agility with continuous yells of support. After twenty minutes of play, the score was nil all. Georges was proud. Once again he had not allowed a single puck to cross him. He smiled with satisfaction.

All of sudden, the fatigue set in, but even worse this time. It felt like daggers were piercing Georges' chest. A chill went up his spine. He wiped the excess sweat from his face with his sleeve as he skated off the ice. Georges looked down at his moist sleeve and noticed a crimson stain. He glared at this arm and wiped his face again. The red mark grew larger. "Mon Dieu!" He was bleeding. But where was it coming from? He wasn't hit during the first period. He felt a trickle from his mouth and tasted iron. Georges realized he was bleeding from his mouth.

Georges' pale face was even whiter than usual. His teammates and coach stared at him with concern when he walked into the dressing room with his bloody sleeve. Coach Léo Dandurand rushed over to where is sat down to rest. "Georges, you don't look so good," he said gravely. "Are you all right?"

"I'm fine, I'm fine," Georges replied coolly.

Then Léo uttered words that Georges had never heard before in his fifteen years with the Canadiens, "Maybe you should take it easy and sit out the second period."

Georges used all of his strength to jump up and exclaimed, "Quoi? Are you kidding? I'm perfectly all right. I don't need to rest. Didn't you see how well I played in the first period? If I was sick, don't you think I would have let in a few goals? This is ridiculous. I've played with many more injuries than this. I've never missed a game before, and I don't intend on missing this one. Coach, you know that a little blood can't stop me." He paused briefly and continued, "Besides, the team and the fans are counting on me. I can't let them down."

"Well, if you insist. Are you sure you're okay?" asked Léo after Georges' passionate soliloquy.

"Trust me. I'm fine."

The intermission passed by quickly. Georges felt a little better after sitting down those twenty minutes.

Second period began with the Habs winning the first face-off again. Georges stood in position at the goalie crease focusing on the action. He tried to concentrate on the game in front of him but could not ignore the pain within him anymore. Within the first few minutes of the period, his vision started to get blurry. He blinked a couple of times, but it did not help. Georges was feeling light-headed, and the arena around him started to spin. The next thing he could remember was everything going dark.

The game stopped abruptly. Teammates skated towards Georges' limp body lying on the ice. Everyone in the crowd rose to their feet with worried expressions. For the first time throughout the whole game, Mt. Royal Arena was silent.

"Georges! Georges!" Léo yelled as he made his way to the net. "Are you okay?" No response. "Georges! Can you hear me?" But it was futile; his star goalkeeper just lay lifeless. Georges' teammates slowly picked him up in unison and somberly carried him off the ice.

Groggily, Georges opened his eyes and stared in confusion. He could not remember where he was, what he was doing or what happened. The trainer stood over Georges examining his body with a hand on his forehead. "Monsieur, do you have any chest pains?" Before Georges could answer, the trainer remarked to someone else in the room, "He's burning up. He's got a temperature of 105. This man needs to get to a hospital immediately!"

At the hospital, the first few words out of the doctor's mouth were what Georges had feared the most for the past couple of weeks. He had an aching suspicion of what might have been causing his severe discomfort. He had tried to avoid it and prayed to God it was nothing. "Out of sight, out of mind," he thought. He hid it from his wife, children, friends and teammates so he could keep playing, but it was inevitable.

The doctor affirmed, "La tuberculose." The dreaded tuberculosis – Georges' heart sank. "I'm afraid it appears to be quite advanced," continued the doctor. "I'm sorry," he touched George's shoulder.

On that day, November 28, 1925, after playing for sixteen seasons, 328 consecutive games, winning three championships, including two Stanley Cup wins, with the Montréal Canadiens, Le Concombre de Chicoutimi was forced to retire involuntarily.

The next couple of months were agonizing for Georges and his teammates. Georges asked to repose in his hometown, Chicoutimi. The Habs were playing disastrously as they could not stop worrying about their star goalie.

Georges visited his teammates one last time to try to calm their nerves and say goodbye. He arrived at the arena the time he would have had he been playing. His uniform and equipment were laid out for him. The players stared in disbelief. Was this the same man they knew and loved? He was so pale that he could have been a ghost. His thin body looked frail, like it would crumble to pieces at the first touch. His eyes lacked the fervor and enthusiasm they were accustomed to. Instead, there stood an old, sickly man with sullen eyes and a gaunt face. Georges barely made eye contact. He nodded in recognition and whispered, "Good luck." He reached for his prized blue and red jersey, the one he wore when they won their last Stanley

Cup in '24. He grabbed it and slowly walked away without staying for the game to begin.

Four months after collapsing on the ice, at age 39, Georges Vézina passed away.

The once powerful Habs performed poorly that season and did not make it to playoff contention.

To commemorate their star goalie, the owners of the Canadiens decided to present a trophy to the NHL during the 1926-27 season, aptly named the Vézina Trophy. To this day, the NHL annually awards the prestigious trophy to the "goalkeeper adjudged to be the best at this position."

This fictionalized account is based on actual events.

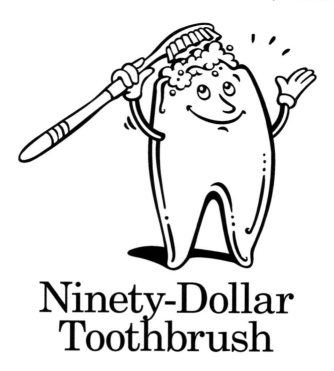

Ninety-Dollar Toothbrush

By Mort Laitner

I am comfortably sitting in a cavernous auditorium at our annual educational conference. The speaker is our health department dentist: a driller of children's mouths and minds. She gives us a modified version of the talk she gives third graders. Being orally fixated (I am an attorney), I listen intently as she describes the best brushing techniques.

"Brush them horizontally, in circular motions." she teaches. "Don't forget to brush your tongue."

Touching my thumbnail to my lower lip, I ponder, that's the way I brushed as a kid, but my current hygienist taught me to brush vertically. The hygienist explained, "To get those food particles out of the cracks between your teeth the bristles have a better chance of entry if you brush vertically." And she never taught me to brush my tongue.

Next the health department dentist explains the virtues of flossing. She continues, "You know the yellowish, sticky paste that accumulates on you teeth that's called plaque? Brushing and flossing removes the plaque and acids that build up in your mouth. These acids destroy gums."

Years ago, my current hygienist converted me into a flosser by showing me glossy photos of horrifying reddened, bloody gums and talking about gum disease. She warned, "Do you want to lose your teeth! You're starting to show signs of periodontal disease-gingivitis." She put a mirror in front of my mouth. "I have to set another appointment with you for the periodontal cleaning, and we will have to do the Tetracycline gum line injections. It is going to be painful, but we have to get this condition corrected so that your gums will stop receding." She said.

"Yikes, my gums are bleeding and swollen!" I exclaimed. "I don't want my gums to recede. I cherish my smile. What do I do?"

She replied, "Commence the practice of daily oral hygiene. Brush and floss after meals, and buy this Oral-B toothbrush." The Oral-B magically appeared before my eyes in a magnificently designed box. She explained, "It comes with its own computer-chip brain which announces to your hand and mouth when it's time to change quadrants. The modulating speed on the brush head changes every thirty seconds."

I advise her, "I hardly ever brush for more than a minute."

"Buddy, those days are over. Do you want me to show you those pictures again?"

"Please, no, once was enough." I whimpered. "How much does the Oral-B cost?"

"Ninety dollars." she nonchalantly responded.

I wondered how much commission she got for each electric toothbrush.

I queried, "Do you take MasterCard? The most I ever spent on a brush was $3.98, and I thought I was a big spender."

Now the hygienist was silent.

I thought: No teeth, no smile, and no fun. I continued this horror movie: gingivitis, gum disease, bad breath, and nightmares of scary dental surgery. Suddenly $90 bucks seemed cheap.

"I'll take it!" I exclaimed. "I promise I'll use it."

Back in the auditorium, listening to the dentist reiterating the best brushing practices, I visualize my morning ritual. I am in front of my Dell—mindlessly playing minesweeper—my Oral-B vibrating away for 5 minutes. One computer in front of me having stolen my brain, while another pulsates in my mouth cleaning my tongue and teeth. Every 30 seconds I am brought back to reality by the brush-time quadrant continuum.

I hear the auditorium resonate with applause for our dentist. As I clap, I think of the MasterCard commercial:

Toothpaste, $3
Oral-B Toothbrush, $90
A healthy mouth...priceless

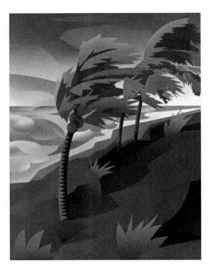

Hurricane

By Tracie Dickerson

"News flash! IKE has now been upgraded to a category 3 Hurricane."

The words scroll across my TV set. I sit on the edge of my couch, terrified.

The storm has started to make an upward turn. My heart sinks as I picture my family, friends and home in Galveston. I wonder if this 730 mile wide monster is the "big one." We're overdue. I hold my breath as childhood memories wash over me.

I was five years old covered with super itchy mosquito bites. My mom said to me, "Alicia is coming."

I innocently asked, "Who is Alicia?"

Mom explained, "Alicia is not a who. She's a hurricane."
"Mom, is she a bad one?"

My mother cautiously replied, "We'll see honey. Don't worry about this storm. We're tough Texans. We can take it."

I didn't understand the panic in her tone, and I didn't know why we put big X's on our windows with masking tape.

By the next day those mosquito bites turned into chicken pox. I would like to think my mom would have wanted to break family tradition and leave the island for the Category 3 storm.

But the evacuation orders came too late. By the time the mayor ordered, "Leave the island immediately. Go to the shelters!" the bridge was impassable and the ferries had closed.

There was no choice but to stay as the storm pushed ashore. We were supposed to go to our shelter; but it was impossible to leave. Nervous shelter workers driving a shuttle came to pick us up. They risked their lives to save Mom and me from this monster. When they arrived, Mom honestly told them, "My daughter has chicken pox."

They politely responded, "Ma'am, I'm sorry to tell you but kids with chicken pox are not allowed in shelters."

Mom answered, "I understand. Thanks for your courage and effort. God bless you." Then I heard the wind slam the screen door as workers ventured back into the storm.

I remember the way the sky looked. The fear that a pre-hurricane sky put into me was indescribable. I knew something bad was about to happen. The entire sky turned dark and foreboding. I realized that shelter shuttle had been our last hope.

The winds had become too strong to drive. We couldn't get to my grandparents' house, so we hid in our hall closet that my mom made into a camping oasis. Somehow she scrunched in a mattress, herself, itchy me, an eighty-pound dog, some food and water in a closet that was only about four feet across and not very deep.

As we sat in the closet I heard the wind whip through our house and I thought about another family hurricane story when my mom was a little kid. My grandmother heard the winds start, and she went into take care of my mother and my aunts. My grandmother was frightened, and because of her fear, her children also became scared. My grandfather slept soundly the entire night. When he awoke the next morning, he queried, "Why is everyone so tired and cranky?"

I thought to myself storms lead to panic so try stay calm for Mom's sake.

Then the power went out. In total darkness, with my dog crushing me I whispered, "Mom, are you okay?"

She replied, "Yes baby, I'm okay .This will be over soon. Don't worry."

Sometimes my mom would open the door to go check on things. I admired her courage and asked, "What is going on out there?

She said, "Tracie, it's almost over; just a little more time. We're doing fine. This old house is a survivor."

Eventually, the storm subsided. Or so I thought. It was fun to finally get to go outside. The weather was beautiful. I did not understand that there was not a lot of time before the other side of the eye would come, but I remember how quiet everything was. My neighbors talked about the calm before the storm. Maybe it was the calm during the eye. I was too young to understand, but I watched as all of the neighbors gathered and did things in a panic. Hammers, ladders, boards – it was a world wind. Before I knew it, (and with a lot of whining) we were back in the closet. For awhile the phone worked, and I recall listening to the radio announcing the dangers of the storm while I scratched my itchy pox. At some point, the radio died, and I heard the wind whipping around the house. Once in awhile, my mom and I would take a look out of the window where one of the boards had a knot that left a peep hole. I saw lightening, tornadoes, and a green sky.

My mom was always looking at the backyard. Later that day, during the storm, we heard a deafening, ripping and cracking noise. We prayed together. And as we prayed I remembered a story my grandfather told me about my great-grandmother and her family's survival through the 1900 storm.

My grandfather described that the 1900 storm killed over 6000 people, and it came with no warning. The weatherman for the island knew there was a problem, but his hands were tied by Washington. All weather reports were required to go through them. Also, Cuba tried to warn us the hurricane was coming, but just a few days before, the federal government stopped weather communications with Cuba.

The days leading up to the storm were perfect. There were few clouds in the sky. Everyone enjoyed playing at the beach. On the day of the storm, the weather started out beautiful, but quickly began to turn.

Before they knew it, the water began to rise as the sky became dark. My family went into their homes, and the water began to come in under the doors, and up through the floorboards. Eventually the water pressure was too much for the windows, and the panes began to explode. Water flowed into the house. The family had retreated into the attic to escape the ever rising waters. Water then began to flood the attic. My great-great grandfather took an axe and started chopping a hole in the roof so they could escape from drowning. After telling me this story, my grandparents would point to doors in the roofs of houses. Even today, my attic has two small windows, and there is an axe at the top of the stairs. Eventually Alicia passed, and we ventured out. I recollect only one thing. The hundred year-old oak tree had toppled over. It knocked down four fences. My mom told me the loud noise we heard was the tree falling,and the loud branches snapping as it toppled over. I will never know why it fell in the exact opposite direction of the wind; but had it followed the wind, this forty-foot tree would have fallen onto our house, and my mother, my dog and I would have met an untimely demise.

As I see TV pictures of Ike's destruction of Galveston 's seawall which is covered in debris, I wonder about my family, friends and home. When I hear stories of the search and rescue missions and the recovery of the dead, I think about my aunt's cousin, who panicked leaving the safety of his home to later drown in his car.

Today, I reflect about the life lessens that my family has taught me:

Don't panic during a storm

Show courage to your loved ones so they won't panic.

AND NEVER FORGET TO BE PREPARED.

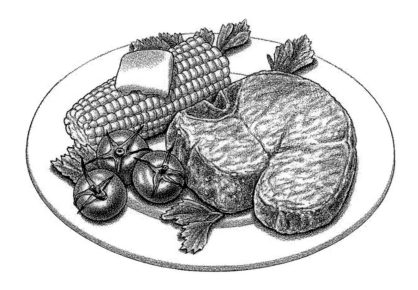

Signs

By Mort Laitner

I'm sitting on a shellacked wooden bench, typographically pecking away on my butter laden corn-on-the-cob. My wannabe-nutritionist spouse has just mentioned, for the third time, "that corn is soaked in butter!" I give her my award- winning smile of melted-butter-on-fresh-corn-bliss, and I nod in agreement. Her latest comment about the butter made me realize that it was missing a little something. Then I had an epiphany -- to get to corn quintessence; I must sprinkle three shakes of salt for good measure. As some of the salt bounces off and some sinks into the butter, I only faintly hear my wife warning "You don't need to add salt to that corn!" As I closed in on the cob, my mouth watered in greedy anticipation. The bite was everything I had hoped for... and more! Pure bliss. I was instantly transformed to another, younger, more carefree time, a time full of Indian summers.

When I took my second bite, I thought about Kafka who allegedly chewed his food thirty times before swallowing. (Try it you'll surprise your taste buds). He believed it aided his digestion. After ten chews, the kernels liquefy and crawl down my throat. I wash them down with a glass of ice cold water in which a slice of lemon floats. (The lemon aids my digestion) I've promised my doctor I would stop drinking soda to lose weight.

Taking my eyes off my plate, I scan Shorty's décor – lots of old stuff stuck to the walls, like the Jack Daniel's "White Rabbit Saloon" sign (subliminal message to encourage beer drinking) and a Marilyn Monroe tray advertising shampoo. Then a baked enamel sign catches my eye.

No spitting.
Fines $5 to $100
By Order of the Health Department

This sign a reproduction of an early 1900's railway station posting for the prevention of consumption (TB). The scientists of that day thought that saliva on the ground some how entered the body causing the dreaded disease.

I proudly announce to the wife, "That sign seems to be working no one is spitting on the floor. That's the Health Department in action."

She glares at me and responds, "From what planet did you get you sense of humor?" My waitress cradles my plate of baby back ribs and a sweet potato wrapped in tin foil. I remove the foil slicing the potato in half and inserting a glob of butter. I watch the butter convert into steam and float into the air. I smell the rich aroma rising from the ribs. I hear, "You know those ribs will clog your arteries!"

While wrapping my lips onto the meaty bones, I mumble, "Tell me something I don't know." I take a second look at the spitting sign. I think about how the Department markets our health message in restaurants. There is no enamel sign which reads:

Cut your salt intake.
Eat less butter.
Eliminate soft drinks.
Recommended by your Health Department.
We care about you.

Standing in line to pay the cashier, I remember Simon and Garfunkel's lyrics from the Sounds of Silence.

"The message of the prophets is written on the subway walls."

I visualize the health message signs hanging on restaurant walls through out the state.

Flipping a nickel into tin bucket, I retrieve a mini-chocolate mint from the glass jar and hear, "You don't need dessert after that meal!"

As the mint melts in my mouth I say to myself," Sweet idea!" I wonder if I will ever see such signs on eatery walls and whether the message will ever sink in. ☀

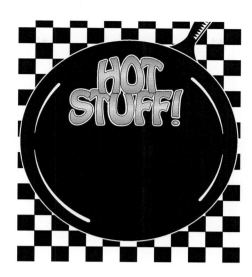

Frying Pan

By Mort Laitner

Pulling the frying pan off the shelf, I glance at its interior surface, a Jackson Pollack in black and silver. Holding the handle I notice for the first time that there is an egg-shaped hole in its base.

I question, "How many years have I used you?"

"Too many to count."

"Did I own you when I started at the health department?"

"We were both young and fully-coated in Teflon innocence."

I continue to study my partially covered friend as I flick a teaspoon of butter into her middle. It melts as quickly as a snow flake hitting the hood of a running car. As the butter liquefies, I inhale the cooking oil's soft scent.

I examine the wounds of a thousand scrapes.

Those were the days before anthrax, bioterrorism attacks and white powder.

Scrape, Scrape, Scrape!

Two yellow pupils surrounded by clear albumin stare back at me
on my whole-wheat toast.

"Look at deep cuts scaring my face."

Those were the days of rabies infected raccoons, psittacosis
carrying parrots, and equine encephalitis!

Abrasion, Abrasion, Abrasion!

This stressed-out-stainless-piece-of-steel has fried thousands of
eggs, bacon strips and sausage patties.

Those were the days of syphilitic babies, AIDS demented heroin
addicts, and persons with tubercular-filled chest cavities.

Scratch, Scratch, Scratch!

My skillet has seen better days; most of its non-stick
coating erased.

Those were the days of freezes, cut backs, and dismissals.

Rub, Rub, Rub!

But after years of use I am one with this DuPont coated product.
My hands repeatedly touch its handle.
I wash and dry her with loving care.
I could not replace it with a new Cuisine de France.

As I gently place the pan back on the shelf, realizing that over
the years the pan's Teflon has etched my veins, becoming part of me
as have all my health department experiences.

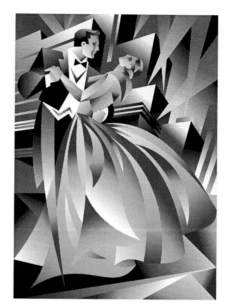

My Worst Crisis

By Tamar Scheinberg

I t was to be the end of my husband's life and my worst crisis. After 43 years together, I watched him go from a positive, healthy husband to a withered man comfortable only when bent forward with his head down. I had witnessed death before with my parents; I knew I would lose them. But losing my husband, Rafi, was different. He was my strength, my rock, and nothing could shake him.

At first, when we found out that he had stage 4 lung cancer, he poured through medical literature. Rafi studied medicine for a year in Argentina, so he looked for alternative treatments before conceding to chemotherapy.

Rafi believed in doctors, medicine, scientific research, and prayed for remission, despite his stage 4 verdict. He smoked for more than 30 years, but the smell of cigarette smoke always bothered him whenever he had a cold. In 1984, during a bad cold, he stopped smoking permanently because of a coughing spell he could not fight off.

When Rafi found out he had cancer, he thought he could beat it. I tried to be optimistic knowing his strength.

He applied for clinical trials and was particularly interested in trying the drug Iressa, which had promising results to patients with lung cancer. The oncologists did not want to "waste time" and started him on chemotherapy. This made him ineligible to participate in clinical trials for new drugs. The chemotherapy deteriorated his health, and he decided to discontinue treatment. There was no radiation therapy available to him. His lungs filled with liquid and were periodically drained.

Through a contact we got in touch with a Hungarian physician involved in research with cancer patients in their final stages. This doctor put us in contact with physicians in Hungary who gave us hope for Rafi's remission.

These treatments were discovered in 1965 when a farmer who had cancer lost his chickens to Newcastle disease, but the farmer miraculously recovered from cancer as his chickens died off. Hungarian scientists then studied the anomaly. They developed the Newcastle vaccine.

We immediately left for Budapest. When Rafi's doctors learned that chemotherapy had no effect on his cancer, he was administered the Newcastle vaccine. We remained in Budapest for a couple of weeks where Rafi was injected with the vaccine on a daily basis and returned to Miami with additional doses. While we were in Budapest, we rarely left our rental apartment, as it was difficult for him to walk and climb steps. On those rare occasions when we ventured out, the summer weather was heavenly. We strolled along the banks of the Danube and savored the dark, rich sweetness of Hungarian pastries. While Rafi watched soccer on television, I toured without him.

Rafi continued to take the vaccine we brought back, although it was now given to him by his oncologist directly through his port hole as opposed to injections. The oncologist did not think the vaccine would be viable but went along with it to please Rafi.

When the amount that we brought back finished, we were informed that the vaccine was no longer in production. We learned a Dutch company was developing a similar vaccine; however, it would take months before we could get more of it. We discovered the Newcastle vaccine was used in the U.S. mainly for chickens, but some patients with Mesothelioma received the vaccine and had been in remission for several years.

Rafi's tumor shrank, but the fluid in his lungs continued to recur and had to be removed every two weeks. Unfortunately, during the fluid removal process, pneumothorax occurred, and one lung was punctured and collapsed.   I watched my beloved Rafi fight his physicians to try to restore his lung, but it was impossible. After this, Rafi gave up hope.

He suffered during the final stages of his life. He refused further treatment. His only comfortable position was sitting in a chair bent forward with his head down.   He signed himself into hospice. From that point on he was only administered oxygen and morphine.

My son flew in from Israel. We took turns sitting with him. Morphine did the job quickly and efficiently, as it had with my mother. Within three days, Rafi fell into a coma. A few hours later he was gone.

The light of my life died. Forty-three years of matrimony, for better or for worse, through good times and bad, through sickness and health. I knew I had to move on, but the months that followed were grueling.

During the grieving process my life collapsed: my daughter divorced, my dog was put to sleep, and I sold my house. I needed to make a new future. I moved to Fort Lauderdale to be closer to my family. I joined Hadassah, a women's service organization and made new friends. Hadassah became my security blanket. I watched my grandson grow into a fine, young, strong man. My daughter found a new love.

My life moved on but my companion, my love and my best friend, Rafi, remains with me always. His death was not my end. ⚜

Tamar Scheinberg is a world traveler who now resides in Broward County, Florida.

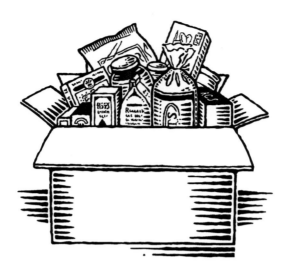

Living in America

By JD Shingles

On Saturday, I was going to purchase a 10 lb. bag of rice from BJ's for the Haitian Food Drive. But, a strange thing happened while I was there. I placed a bag of rice into my shopping cart and briskly walked towards the checkout. Feeling peaceful and happy, I caught myself humming one of James Brown's tunes, "I Feel Good". You know, the song that goes something like this:

"Whoa-oa-oa! I feel good, duh nuh nuh nuh nuh nuh
I knew that I would, now
I feel good, I knew that I would,
now so good, so good, I got you ,dooh doo doo dooh."

Suddenly, I felt warm. I could not pinpoint it, but I was elated. Yes! This warm sensation came over me because I was helping the less fortunate.

My mind reverted to the song –
"Whoa! I feel nice,
like sugar and spice,
I feel nice, like sugar and spice,
so nice, so nice,
I got you, yeah."

Then my warmth began to take on a deep chill. My body froze. I quickly turned my head from side-to-side. Curiously, I surveyed my surroundings looking for somebody; anybody. I stared intently at the lifeless bag of rice in my shopping cart.

"Ok. JD, it's a bag of rice; rice can't make you stop dead in your tracks."

Then, from out of nowhere, a funky voice began to speak to me.

"Do you really feel good?" said the Voice. I clutched my cart's handrail tighter as perspiration began to trickle down my arms and brows. "Do you really feel good?" the Voice repeated. My eyes, once again, scanned my surroundings, but no one was in sight.

The Voice and I were in a dog fight. The Voice chuckled as it leaned forward and whispered in my ear, "Yes. You can do better?" Hastily, I wheeled my shopping cart around and went back to pick up a second bag of rice.

Now I was back in line, just two shopping carts away from the cashier. The Voice returned. It spoke softly, "JD, you live in America; help me out, you live in America; eye to eye, station to station, hand to hand, across the nation. I broke out in a feverish sweat. Oh, no! "What's going on, here"? The purpose for my trip to BJ's was to purchase a bag of rice to donate to the Food Drive. The Voice reminded me that I live in America. And, for centuries America has been the world's ambassador.

I went back to the aisle and got a third bag of rice. "This is it! I do not care what the Voice says."

I dashed to checkout as the Godfather of Soul lyrics continued to play in my head.

After checking out, James' voice vanished.

As strange as this may seem, the hardest working man in show business challenged me to fulfill a hunger's harvest.

I live in America.

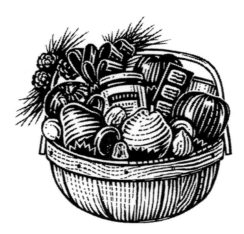

The Love Basket

By Jessie Bellevue

Our West Perrine Women Infant and Children (WIC) team wanted to honor a needy family for Christmas. After much discussion, we chose a lovely mentally challenged mother of four.

We collected canned beans, fruits and vegetables, boxes of pasta and hot chocolate from our kitchen cabinets and put together them in a basket. We wrapped the basket with red and green foil and candy-cane ribbons.

We knew our client took the bus for her appointments and it would be easier if a family member with a car drove the goodies back to her home. So we called her mom and said, "You don't know us but we work of the Health Department. We would like to help your daughter and her kids with a Christmas basket this holiday."

"WOW!" Grandma replied, "How can I help?

"If you could please give your daughter and her children a ride to the clinic on December 15, it would help."

"Please don't mention this to your daughter. We would like to make it a surprise," we whispered.

Grandma loved the surprise idea. She proceeded to tell us of a tale of the absent father of the first two children, the abuse which resulted in the third pregnancy and the occasional help given by the father of the fourth child. She also mentioned her other daughter who had an 18 month old baby and had stopped receiving WIC benefits. She added that they could not afford to celebrate Christmas.

After hearing such a dismal story, we decided to bring Christmas to them. A nonprofit organization donated toys for the children, and we bought small gifts for the three adults.

The family arrived at 1 PM, and we presented them with the food basket and gifts. The adults cried tears of gratitude. The children became wide-eyed and smiles broke out of their faces. We also used this opportunity to certify four of the children into the WIC program for another year.

They were overjoyed. We cheered up a family in need and the happiness multiplied to each and every one of us.

Throughout the year we at WIC help those in need feed their families and during this holiday season we not only provided them with bundles of food but with a basket of love.

Jessie Belview is an employee of the Miami-Dade County Health Department's Women, Infants and Children (WIC) program.

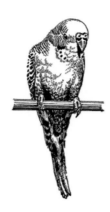

Blessings Can Help

By Lori Jordahl

"There was domestic violence in my house this morning!" You could hear the gasps….

"The baby almost died and would have, if I hadn't been there!" Now, you could hear a pin drop….

The crowd of over 100 participants in a workshop on AIDS and Women were leaning forward to hear the next words…**"So if you hear a cheep, cheep, it's my baby parakeet, I got him just in time."** Sighs reverberated around the room.

I used this real time experience to get my audience's attentioni and to lead my talk on the importance of prevention, communication and seeking assistance. It was after all, the early '90's and AIDS Prevention was still a fairly new topic, especially when it came to women. If only we paid attention and really took action then. Now, years later, women are still too afraid, unsure, unbelieving or have not learned that they are important and can help make a difference.

After the workshop, which included some emotional disclosures from participants, insightful questions and well wishes for the baby parakeet, I did what every good mother would do. I went into the ladies room to get hot water, mix the formula and feed the baby.

The parakeets in my nest hatched out of their shells at different intervals. This little guy, the last born, with hardly a feather was being pecked to death by siblings trying to get more of the food. I had to save him that morning, it couldn't wait!

So, in the ladies room while I was putting droplets of food down his beak, a group of Ministers approached me from the Balm In Gilead*. They had been in my workshop and were not only moved by my story but how I incorporated it into AIDS Prevention messages. **I had tears in my eyes as they circled around me and blessed us.**

That was the first 2 blessings that came from this bird. But there were more to come. My friend and colleague, Ellen, was so moved by this experience and a chance to hold the baby that she asked me if I had any hand raised babies that she could have. With a smile in my heart, I told her I would be delighted to give her one and did so the very next day. Her friends and staff hearing that she was getting a pet all chided me for entertaining her with this craziness.

Ellen and "Buddy" were my third blessing. She opened her heart and home, spoiling this parakeet for many years. They made my family smile every time we received pictures and cards for Buddy's birth family.

Speed ahead more than 10 years... I am presenting a poster session at the same National Conference. Two ladies approached me with comforting eyes and large smiles. They told me I probably wouldn't remember them, but I had made a difference in their lives, and they hoped that I was still raising parakeets.

These 2 Ministers reminded me, that blessings no matter how big or small, are still blessings. My work in Public Health is a Blessing. I make a difference!

P.S. Don't you know that when I left the conference that afternoon, I made a stop...and arrived home with 4 new little parakeets! ☼

*Reference: **The Balm In Gilead, Inc.**™ is a not-for-profit, non-governmental organization whose mission is to improve the health status of people of the African Diaspora by building the capacity of faith communities to address life-threatening diseases, especially HIV/AIDS.

Lori Jordahl is an author and an employee the Miami-Dade County Health Department's Sexually Transmitted Diseases division.

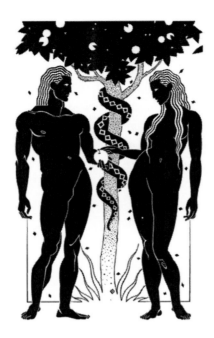

Why Snakes?

By Mort Laitner and Amy Tejirian

May 2008

"I'm so excited! We've completed editing *Healthy Stories* 2008, and it's ready to go to the publishers," Mort exclaimed as he walked out of his office holding a stack of papers.

In unison, Tracie and Heather breathed a sigh of relief. All those months of writing and editing had finally paid off – a book with twenty-five original stories and seven stories from the original book translated in Spanish and Creole. They grinned at each other and headed back to their desks.

Amy took the stack of papers from Mort's hand and started thumbing through it. "Wow, it looks fantastic."

"Thanks," Mort replied. "But I think that something is missing. I can't put my finger on it. When it pops in my head, I'll know."

There was a brief pause. Amy handed the stack of papers back to Mort and started to head back to her desk when she heard Mort yelled, "Eureka! We need a logo."

Amy turned around, "That's a good idea. Have any ideas of what the logo should look like?"

"Come into my office and help me brainstorm," Mort said motioning his arm towards his office.

Amy sat at Mort's computer while Mort started to think out loud, "We need something that represents health, but is unique. We want something eye-catching. It should be colorful, yet simple."

Amy listened attentively while she surfed the net. "That sounds like a handful. How can we do all that in a little logo?" As she asked the question, she googled "health" in images. "Maybe we can get some kind of idea looking at other pictures of health."

However, Mort did not hear a word she said. He was deep in his thoughts. His eyes were focused on another familiar logo, the Miami-Dade County Health Department's smiling apple. "Eureka!" He exclaimed for the second time in ten minutes. Before Mort could continue, Amy quipped, "You're a regular Archimedes today."

"Snakes!" stated Mort as his eyes lit up.

"Snakes? Why snakes?" Amy was utterly confused.

Mort answered, "Ever hear of Genesis, Adam and Eve, the apple and of course the snake?"

"Um, yeah," Amy said hesitantly, "but what does that have to do with our book?" She continued googling images. This time her search term was "health snake". Immediately a couple of pictures appeared of a short herald's staff entwined by two snakes in the form of a double helix. "Oh, look, the caduceus, the symbol commonly used for medicine or doctors. I guess snakes do have something to do with health, but what?"

"Quite ironic!" Mort retorted, "Since in Roman iconography the Caduceus was carried in the left hand of the Greek god Hermes, the messenger of the gods, guide of the dead and protector of merchants, gamblers, liars and thieves."

"The symbol has neither connection with Hippocrates nor any association with the healing arts."

"How about that other snake health symbol?"

Amy asked, "What other snake symbol?" She clicked the mouse on another image that resembled the last one but was a little different.

It linked her to the website for the American Medical Association. "This one?" She pointed to the computer screen.

"Yup, that's the one - the rod of Asclepius, the one with the herald's staff which carries only one snake and no wings," Mort responded

"Well, it has the blessing of the American Medical Association."

"Funny you should mention that, the AMA used the caduceus until 1912 when they prudently switched to the rod of Asclepius."

Amy started to get frustrated. "You still haven't answered my question. Why snakes? What does that have to do with our book?"

"OK, OK, I'll tell you. Ever hear of Hygeia, Greek goddess of health?"

"Nope but I'll bet I'll get an ear full about her. I can Google her if you want. How do you spell that?"

"I'm not sure but it should be spelled similarly to hygiene." replied Mort. "Do a Wikipedia search for her."

Amy tried the best she could to spell the unfamiliar word in the search box. Her guess was correct because a page about the Greek goddess Hygieia or Hygeia appeared. They both scanned the screen for a few minutes absorbing all the information they could about this figure in Greek mythology.

Mort broke the silence, "Originally, she was the goddess of physical health and later became the goddess of mental health. Hygeia was often symbolized with a snake drinking from a cup. The snake was associated with healing. It's from Hygeia we get the word hygiene. Hygiene is the science of preserving health. And that, my dear, is why *Healthy Stories* uses snakes in its logo; health departments are all about preserving health."

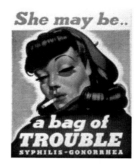

A Bag of Trouble

By Morton Laitner

I'm standing on the Mall in the nation's capitol, staring in amazement at the Washington Monument, when I glance at a light pole securing a colorful advertisement. It reads, "See 'An Iconography of Contagion,' exhibit at the National Academy of Sciences."

I'm traveling with my youngest son, Blake, on his way back to university. I know these are the days he and I will never forget. Days that bond a father and son as tightly as memories glued into a photo album.

"Blake, how about being good to the old man, let's go study public health art and contagion at the Academy?"

"Sure Dad, I'd love to learn about contagious diseases," he sarcastically replied.

As we stroll across the National Mall, I grasp why my eyes focused on that colorful banner. Her silhouette was angelically framed in white, a sultry brunette wearing a red beret. As the traffic whizzed by, I realized the picture held my hidden passion for French women wearing red crepe hats and smelling of imitation Chanel No. 5, cheap champagne and stale tobacco. This beauty's glossy full-colored red lips perfectly matched the red beret resting lazily on her head.

Blake comments, "Dad, there's another banner with that hooker on it."

"Son, thanks for pointing it out, I want to see what it says." I read out loud,

"She may be... a bag of TROUBLE---SYPHILIS-GONNORHEA."

I think short, sweet and to the point.

Blake exclaims, "Dad, that's gross!"

I explain, "Son, that's a World War II poster designed to keep American soldiers from procuring the services French prostitutes. To American GI's, Frenchie was a symbol of danger and death."

Blake studied the drawing and exclaimed, "What a mixed message!

They show a hot French babe and tell Army boys, who are about to risk their lives in battle, stay away because she "MAY" be a bag of trouble. Why didn't they have another poster with a condom on it saying, she is not a bag of trouble if you use one of these."

I laughed as I rested my hand on Blake's shoulder and said, "You know, back when you were born, condom posters were verboten."

Pausing I continued, "I remember how difficult it was in the 80's during the beginning of the AIDS crisis. How appalled state representatives were when we released condom posters. The image of Captain Condom injected fear in fun-loving Florida.

"Dad, are you suggesting health officials sometimes bow to the pressures of political correctness?", said Blake.

"Blake, there is a life lesson to be learned here. We who serve the people walk a fine line between protecting health and not offending the vox populi. I sighed, "That my son, is the real **BAG OF TROUBLE.**"

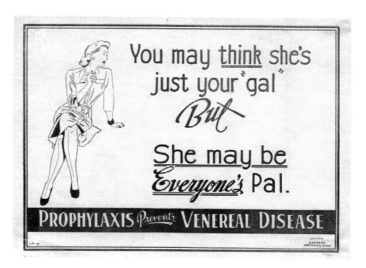

Prophylaxis

By Mort Laitner

WWII, 1944, somewhere in the lower forty eight, a young mid-western illustrator is given a war assignment.

His boss barks out the order, "Draw me a young innocent woman who may be a tramp!"

Artist thinks out loud, "Tough assignment - a true contradiction." The artist meekly asks, "Boss, do we have the by-line?"

The boss snarls, "Yea, 'You may think she's your 'gal' but she may be everyone's pal.'"

The illustrator knows the US Army is paying his salary. His poster should get soldiers to wear protection-like helmets protecting their heads. Public Health enters the fray, but will it promote trust between the sheets?

The kid imagines a bedroom scene with his girlfriend looking up and asking, "Don't you trust me?" He shakes his head trying to figure out how he would respond.

He queries, "Boss you got any suggestions?"

"Yea, put some lipstick on her and put her legs in nylons with the seam in the middle of each leg."

The boss, starting to enjoy himself, adds, "Make sure her legs are crossed, the skirt is knee length and pose her arm like she's holding a cigarette but don't put one in her hand."

"Thanks, boss great advice, any jewelry on her?"

"Kid, don't over do it. Keep it simple. Just one wrist bracelet. We want to show her angel and devil side."

Three hours later the illustrator carries in his finished product. He proudly lays the sketch on the boss' desk.

"Kid, you have done it! It's a masterpiece! Is she or isn't she fooling around?

This will keep those soldiers guessing. We may not be medics, but I think we just saved a few lives!"

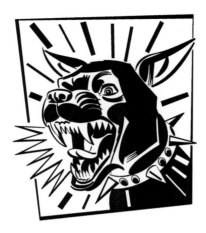

The Shepherd

By Phil Reichert

I saw the postman approaching my home. My neighbor's German shepherd made the same observation. The shepherd charged across the unfenced yard. Faster than Jessie James, the mailman drew his holstered mace and at pistol-drawing level, sprayed the liquid into the dog's eyes. Upon contact, Max yelped louder than a hungry baby. Max rubbed his paws into his reddened eyes as he commenced his retreat. I felt sorry for Max. He was protecting his turf. Today, as I remember that postal carriers were not the only government workers facing attacking canines, my eyes tear. Health department employees aren't even given a canister of mace.

I spent several years doing field work for the sexually transmitted disease program, known simply in the early 1980's as the "VD Program." I had my share of barking-biting dogs. Even Chihuahuas, in their own minds, morph into pit-bulls when a stranger intrudes on their territory. Dogs protect their masters from intruders just as VD Investigators protect their masters from the smorgasbord of sexually transmitted diseases.

My colleague and fellow VD Investigator, Lisa, was deathly afraid of barking dogs in yards. Our duties require serving VD exposure notices to someone who may need testing and treatment...even when the house or apartment was protected by dogs. When there were sonorous pups that kept her from her appointed task, Lisa would return to the office and ask me to accompany her.

One day Lisa asked me to accompany her to a house with three dogs. She had been to the house earlier and decided she could not bring herself to step into the yard with the little yappers. When we pulled up to the house, I saw that the house had a chain-link fence and, yes, three small barking dogs. Even though their barks were loud, none looked as if they could do much damage if they got close enough to bite. If challenged, I was certain these mutts would back down. As I looked at the pups, I gave her a slightly disgruntled look saying, "What! You're afraid of three dogs that would lose a fight against a dying hamster?"

Lisa replied, "But, you're here, and I would hate for one of them to bite me." So, I opened the gate, stepped into their tiny tea-cup territory, and I shuffled to the door. The subject of the contact letter shooed the pups away and listened to what I had to say. As it turned out, the fearless dogs had protected their master temporarily from the news of his exposure, but my news sheparded him to the VD clinic for a penicillin shot and protection from syphilis.

A couple of months later, I was doing field work alone and found an address that was several miles out in the country, the home of another of our VD clients in need of some medication. I pulled up into a long, dirt driveway and opened my car door only to be greeted by one of the largest, most dangerous-looking (and sounding) German shepherds I had ever encountered.

A little history: When I was eight years old, a very large German Shepherd (when you're eight years old, they're all large) chased me down the street while I was riding my bicycle. I remember thinking that I could easily out-pedal the monster dog. Well, I learned that day German shepherds can run pretty darn fast. With his deep, truculent bark, he was gaining on me. In fact, he caught me, clamped down on my ankle and drew blood. He finally gave up when I refused to go down. But I kept pedaling for my life, tears running down my cheeks as I headed home.

Out in the country I looked at what seemed the direct descendant of the shepherd that bit me, and I understood why Lisa preferred to have someone with her when a pooch interrupted her field work. I had driven so far and spent so much time trying to find this STD client, I didn't want to leave without having first delivering my message. Like the hero in an old western movie, I decided to leave the protection of my car and head for the door of the house. I knew I would draw fire from the dog the whole way. My only hope was to get to the door and to the safety of the porch without loosing too much blood. My heart was pounding in my chest as I opened the gate and started for the door, but I figured owner would call off his dog when he saw me moving toward his door in an official looking manner. I glanced down at my Health Department ID and for a moment thought I saw a glittering gold star shining back at me.

I made it to the safety of the porch, and breathless, I knocked on the door. In a few seconds the German Shepherd, teeth glaring, would be at my feet. Of course, no one was home. I drew the paperwork out of my pocket and left it in the doorjamb. Then I whipped around to assess my retreat. I realized I would now have to make it back to my car without the protection I was counting on. The dog followed me to the gate barking with a vengeance every step of the way. Each time the dog would try to take a bite of my leg, he would stop with his snout in the country dirt. Interestingly, he never got closer than about twelve inches from taking a bite out of one of my ankles. I had been all set to kick and punch, to fight my way to the end, but Cujo must have figured that barking loudly usually drove away intruders. Knowing that I had done my duty to protect the person who had been unknowingly exposed to a VD, I returned my sheparding duty to the homeowner's best friend. I hopped back into my car, heart racing, and I drove into the sunset with a good feeling about having helped the community contain another STD and with a new-found empathy for Lisa's feelings about barking dogs. ☼

Philip E. Reichert, MPH is the program administrator of the Hepatitis Prevention Program for the Department of Health in Tallahassee, Florida.

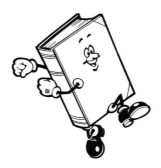

Healthy Stories at the Book Fair

By Tracie Dickerson

We couldn't believe our eyes when the stall directly across from our Healthy Story booth said "My Days with the Doors and other Stories". We had just published a story entitled "People are Strange" and this coincidence was just as odd. Another strange fact was that John Holmes, the author of our story was driving down from Palatka to attend the book fair. John being a major Doors fan, couldn't believe "the Fifth Door" Doug Lubahn who had played bass on four of The Doors' albums, including Strange Days, Waiting for the Sun, and the Soft Parade would be sitting directly across from him all weekend. The night before, John could hardly sleep, thinking about meeting Doug. John carried a copy of his story, which he presented Doug, and they started to reminisce about their lives in the late 60's. They became close enough so that John felt comfortable in asking Doug for a blurb for the back of our next edition. Doug graciously consented to write the following blurb.

"I met John Holmes at the Miami International Book Fair. John related to me his "People are Strange" story, wherein he shared a beer with Jim Morrison. The story just goes to show what an incredible man Morrison was. I know having actually shared a few beers with Jim myself."

Another one of our ideas was to trade *Healthy Stories* with other authors in exchange for their book, and hopefully a blurb from them.

We were quite successful, and have now added to our quarantine library the following editions: The Golden Egg, The Story of Our Miracle Baby, by Debra & Elias Franco; Why Jews Don't Camp, Plus 24 other Hilarious Stories about Everyday Life by Arnie Z. Goldberg; and Breaking up Without Breaking Down, Picking up the Pieces to Become Whole Again by Kristina de la Cal. Not only did we trade for books, but one of our editors succeeded in paying five dollars for an "all-the-books-you-can-carry" deal of the day, that has resulted in an additional forty five books for the Quarantine Exchange Library.

Seeing the Miami-Dade County Health Department banner, many people stopped to take a look at *Healthy Stories*. The Chairman of the Board of County Commissioners, of Miami-Dade County introduced himself after spending some quality time studying our story book. Our medical director, with his whole family, stopped by to say hello! Some health department workers from around the state purchased books as gifts for their colleagues' enjoyment. One patron said, "This is a great idea! Are there any other *Healthy Stories* books in publication in the country?" To which we proudly responded, "No."

One perspective customer yelled to his friend, "Hey look, Miami Dade County Health Department has a book at the book fair!"

But our favorite quote was said by an elderly African-American woman, "The first book I bought at the fair was Obama's, "Audacity of Hope," and the second book was *Healthy Stories*."

Hundreds of readers picked up our *Healthy Stories* bookmarks and business cards. Many of them gave us their e-mail addresses so that we could mail them our new stories. The book fair was a marketing bonanza. Not only did we have fun, we got some street cred. We had the joy of autographing our books in the blistering heat of Saturday and the chill of Sunday. As the parade of ravenous readers marched by our booth, children were magnetically attracted to our book cover, as if by the simple act of touching it would make their own. Readers picked up copies and read a story or two while they decided if *Healthy Stories* would take a place on their bookshelves. Thousands of people saw that the Miami-Dade County Health Department is a community partner.

What a coincidence to find in our story President-Elect Obama, Jim Morrison and the Doors, a golden egg and a beer. How bold. How daring. How audacious.

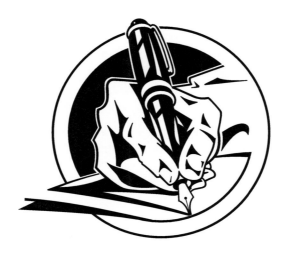

Addicted!

By John Holmes

I am hopelessly hooked. What am I to do now? My addiction has become a part of my life with no end in sight. I have tried to talk to trusted friends, but they just do not understand. I think about it more and more the longer my addiction continues. I am afraid my problem will start to interfere with my daily life if it is not brought under control.

The "monkey" is that I am a first time published author. Just thinking about the possibility of being published again causes lightheadedness and flushing. Where will the next story come from and will it be as good as or better than the last one? I have started several stories since my first one, having yet to get the "fix" to satisfy the craving. You may wonder what the big deal is. Let me put some perspective on this addiction. Many of you reading this are either coffee drinkers or cigarette smokers. What happens if you do not feed your habit daily? What is your mental condition about noontime? What about chocolate? These are personal addictions that only affect you alone. When you are published, the whole world knows. My audience is anyone world wide who can read the English language or has access to the internet. There are people who have read my work in countries whose name I can not even pronounce.

When I drive past a bookstore like Borders, I wonder if any of the people coming out of the store have a copy of my story. I have looked at Amazon.com and have seen *"Healthy Stories"* and my name listed as one of the many fine authors in the book. I noticed that these memories have fed my addiction. My heart rate increases and I perspire. My breathing rate increases, and I start to wonder when the next story line will come to me. I was at another major bookstore this week and was watching the authors with their recently published books talking to their fans. I started thinking about how they must feel when someone purchases a book and requests that they write a short line and sign the book. Those thoughts started my body trembling. I realized that I needed another story or I would go crazy. I now know that what I really need is a book signing tour.

Knowing that a book signing tour is out of the question, I decided to try the next best solution to satisfy my cravings. I purchased a number of issues of *"Healthy Stories"* for family and friends and when I give them each a copy, I have my own book signing moment. It is not the same, but these fans are forever.

There is no way to describe the feeling of being published the first time.

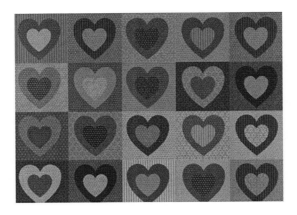

Bittersweet Memories

By Lori Saxon Jordahl

Another World AIDS Day is around the corner, what bittersweet memories... the loss of friends, prayers for an end, and the light of many still passionate about prevention, awareness and helping. My cell phone rings, jolting me out of my thought process. It is my son, Benjamin, my interest was piqued, he never calls from work, so like a good mom, I ask in panic, "Is everything okay?"Benjamin laughs and says, "I was surfing the net and I realized that World AIDS day is next week. So I asked my boss for permission to distribute red ribbons. I was wondering if you could send me some."

A rush of pride flows through my veins as the moment when a loving mom realizes that her child has learned the importance of giving back to the community. I reply, "I'll put them in the mail today. Ben, you made my day. Love you. Bye." I hang up the phone as a filmstrip of memories floods back to me...

First frame: Meeting with the AIDS steering committee in 1989 and deciding we needed to go big: a march down Biscayne Boulevard, a program at Bayfront Park. From there it grew to thousands walking down the Boulevard, singing, chanting and then silence with lit candles. As wax melting down my fingers, I picture the committee's faces and realize that I am the only one still alive.

Second Frame: Protesting with activists costumed as grim reapers ringing bells which tolled for those who collapsed on the sidewalk while others chalked outlines of their bodies.

Third Frame: Feeling goose bumps rise upon hearing the names of family, friends and co-workers called out who have died of AIDS.

Fourth Frame: Looking up at the night sky, staring at the stars Pedro Zamora, The Real World casts and Daisy Fuentes of MTV.

Fifth Frame: Viewing condom commercials from around the world featuring Celia Cruz, Albita, Carmen Electra, Lisa Ray, and Marri Morrow.

Sixth Frame: Tasting my salty tears during candlelight vigils on South Beach-- the ghostly look of faces lit by melting paraffin reflecting their souls as the ocean breeze extinguished their flames.

Seventh Frame: Watching helicopters hang red ribbons on skyscrapers lit by laser light.

Eighth Frame: Smelling burning, dry pinewood from campfires crackling on the beach, rising smoke irritates my tear glands.

Ninth Frame: Shaking my body to hemispheric music, as we dance el tango, el mambo, el meringue, la habanera, and la salsa to express our love of life.

Tenth Frame: Praying, "We open our hearts and minds to the welfare of all people with HIV and AIDS. We ask that they be held in love and feel the Divine support."

Eleventh Frame: Touching the cotton carved letters of The Names Project Quilt, reading tributes to lost loved ones, sewing memories at quilting bees.

Final Frame: Witnessing a one year old boy holding Benjamin's hand as they lit a candle on stage on behalf of children living with AIDS.

I take a moment to reflect on my millisecond mental slide show, and I realize my bittersweet memories of those who have passed on but continue to live in my heart and mind are what drives me. I am glad to know that I have helped my community through this pandemic, and that my work, even in small ways, will live on through people like my son. ☼

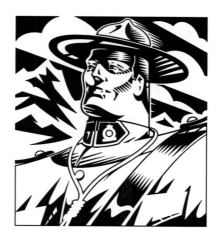

Bad Luck

By Mort Laitner

In the fall of '68, Alan craved leaving the country. He was against the war, feared the draft, and hated studying. Alan followed the hippie trail to the Great White North. It was only a two hour bus ride to the border. He wore his untamed red hair shoulder length. He wore his bell bottoms below his ankles and deep within them he carried a taste for adventure as well as an ounce of Mexican pot. In his back pocket, locked by a metallic button, rested his wallet, which contained his New York State driver's license and one twenty dollar bill.

Alan assured himself he would find an accepting commune in Canada. A place where he would work in exchange for food, drugs and shelter, a lucky new lease on life. He had heard the stories. The bus stopped in a hamlet near the border. He debarked. In the belly of the bus he found his sleeping bag and knapsack. Deep within the sleeping bag he hid his twelve inch Bowie knife with its elk horn handle.

There was a chill hanging in the morning air and low lying dark clouds created a mountain range across the sky. He saw a quaint diner next to the depot. Upon entering "Buck's Coffee and Brew" Alan inquired; "Hey man, how far to the border?"

A farmer wearing a red and green plaid wool hunting cap replied,

"It's about half mile up the road." Alan thought to himself, time for one last cup of American Joe.

A waitress wearing her white apron and a-we-don't-see-many-new-faces smile asked, "How can I help you?"

Alan replied, "Cup of the black stuff -- and if you don't mind, one quick question."

The waitress, "Shoot."

"How hard is it to cross the border?"

The waitress, "No problem, the Canadian Border cops are one hell of a nice bunch of guys. Just don't forget to bring your I.D."

After sipping down the warm brew, Alan paid seventy-five cents for the coffee and left a quarter tip. As he exited the cafe, she chirped, "Thanks and have a safe trip. I'll see you when you come back!"

Alan waved back at her and commenced his half mile trek. "I'm not coming back!" he said contemplating getting set up in his new homeland.

On the hassle-free U.S. side of the border, Alan lied and said he was going to visit relatives in Montreal. Then he entered the Canadian side of the building, the border patrol asked for passports or driver's licenses and proof of financial security. Alan read the large sign on the wall, "SHORT TIME VISITORS ENTERING CANADA MUST POSSESS AT LEAST TWENTY DOLLARS."

Horrified, Alan counted his money. He only had nineteen dollars. Why did he stop for that cup of coffee? He begged the Canadian officials to be made an exception to the rule. Failing to make any head way he cursed out the border security guards with the tongue of a revolutionary war soldier. Glumly he threw his backpack over his shoulder turned south and marched back to the American town. He yelled, ONE LOUSY DOLLAR! WHAT BAD LUCK!

As he walked he felt the presence of a car creeping up behind him. He heard the trumpeting of a siren and turned to look at a squad car with flashing red and blue lights. The auto's loud speaker mounted on the hood blared, "Son, put your hands up in the air and don't make any sudden moves." Alan started shaking. He could not ditch the dope without being seen. The police officer frisked him, found the marijuana and placed him under arrest. Now handcuffed in the back seat of the squad car, Alan longed for the security of his dormitory room. He looked up and saw the waitress staring slack jawed at him from the safety of the diner window. She was right, he thought. He began to weep as he realized his dream of a new life in a new country had turned into a disaster. His head ached as if it was being hammered with a ball pein. He closed his eyes and hallucinated being drug free. Tears rolled down his freckled face he whimpered, "One lousy dollar. What bad luck!" Why me? Why me? Why me?

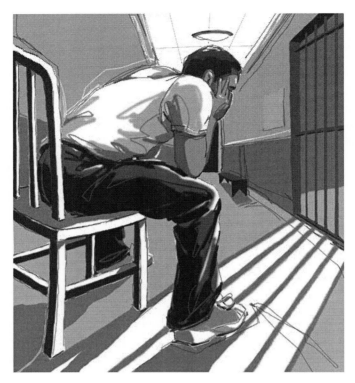

Jail

By Morton Laitner

As Alan sat in his cell, he contemplated suicide. He wondered if the arresting officer found the knife in his sleeping bag. He feared calling his father-- what would he say? His Dad was a loving man, but they grew distant since he left for college. He played out the conversation in his head:

Son: "Dad, please sit down."

Father: His father's voice becoming tenser with each passing word. "Why? Is something wrong?"

Son: "Dad…. I'm in trouble." He pauses, taking a deep breath, and allowing the message to sink in.

Father: "Where are you? What have you done now? Are you in jail?"

Son: "I'm in jail." His voice nervously trembles as he decides to tell his square father why he was arrested, "It is for possession… I…

uh... um... marijuana. I need you to bail me out and I need a ride back to school."

Father: "Are you on acid? You're tripping and you're just messing with my head? Stop it! I knew you I shouldn't have sent you to that college. All those kids get hooked on LSD. You disappointed me too many times! For your sake, I hope this is a joke."

Son: "Sorry, Dad, but this is for real. I need your help. Being locked up is driving me crazy. I got to get out of this cell." He slammed his fist into the iron bars of an adjoining cell causing a trickle of blood to drip on to the white tile floor. "Dad, I need help."

Father: sighs so loud Alan could hear his head shaking. "OK son, I hear you. How much is your bail?"

Son: "One hundred dollars." Tears of relief cascaded down Alan's reddened cheeks as tears of fear ran from his father's eyes onto his lips. His tongue burned as if his tears were made of acid.

Father: "That's a lot of money, I'll have to go to the bank and it will take me about three hours to drive up there and bail you out. Son, hang in there, everything going to be all right." His voice tampered off as Alan heard the phone drop into its cradle.

The police officer escorted Alan in to the hallway, in handcuffs, to a pay phone: asked him for his parent's number, dialed the number for him and upon hearing a voice on the line handed him the receiver.

Alan's Mom was on the line, he immediately asked for his father. "Mom, I need to speak to Dad right now!"

His father got on the line and the call went pretty much as Alan thought.

Alan was escorted back into his cell, where every minute of incarceration seemed like an eternity. He hit his head against the cinder block wall to relieve the pressure occupying his head. After the third bang the external pain grew greater than the internal pressure.

He ran a mind video of the happiest moments in his short life: the women he had loved, his high school friend's playing ball and those acid trips to the other side. Alan closed his eyes and fell asleep on the thin mattress wrapped in a thread bare sheet. He dreamed of Hendrix, Joplin and Morrison. They talked to him.

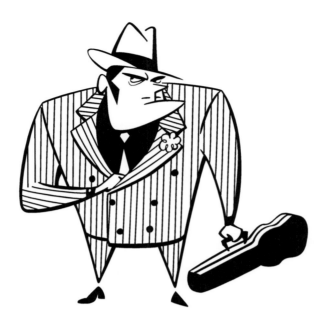

The Godfather

By John Holmes

I'll make you an offer you can't refuse. I'm a big fan of The Godfather saga. Visualize Marlon Brando, "Don Corleone", in his office conducting "Family Business" with a series of amici, friends and associates, requesting favors. The Godfather welcomes them into his magnificently decorated home, offers Chianti, and like "the gentleman" he was, asks of what service he could be. The acquaintance would tell their sad story and after careful thought, the Don would ask his question, "Do you want justice?" Sometimes the amici would say "yes". Sometimes the friend would say something outrageous to which the Godfather would tell them their request was not justice; it was revenge. The Don would then say he would have someone look into the matter and the person would be satisfied with the result. In return, the Don would inquire, "Someday, and that day may never come, I'll call upon you to do justice as a gift on my daughter's wedding day." The wronged person would respond, "Grazie, Godfather."

Much like visitors who asked the Don for favors, I often prayed for guidance. I know my prayers are heard because a few years ago on one terrible night, I got an answer. I was incredibly sick and my future looked bleak. As death approached, I knew I had to do something drastic or I would perish. I needed a plan and fast. I started to see myself in one of those deathbed- salvation scenes. The scene seemed so "Little House on the Prairie". I was not going to go out in a tear jerker moment. As helplessness overtook me, common sense and anger kicked in. My first response was to strike out. My thoughts were of self-pity until I realized that my situation could only be solved by outside intervention. I needed strength tempered with family honor.

All of a sudden, I saw Don Corleone. He tried to tell me something. It seemed so surreal. As morphine partied in my brain, reality became a rare commodity. In my dream, the answers to life's questions appeared. There was no need for me to die. Corleone's lips moved, but I could not hear. I remember begging, "Please speak louder! I can't hear you Godfather!"

His lips moved again "S**** Bl***". I still did not understand. Don Corleone turned and started to walk away. Everything was moving so slow, I could barely breathe when the Godfather turned to me one more time and said "Use your small blessings" and everything went dark.

Several hours later, I awoke. The morphine hallucinations had subsided. There was an eerie feeling inside of me. Haunted memories troubled me. What did Don Corleone mean? Use your small blessings. My thoughts were fixed on Don's message when I saw my family priest walk past my door. I called to him, "Father, do you have a few minutes?" Father Fredo entered my hospital room, full of enthusiasm and understanding. I told him my dream and its unexplained message.

The priest listened attentively and after I completed my story he inquired, "What do you think the dream means?"

WHAT DOES IT MEAN! "I thought you were the expert on blessings. Didn't you learn anything in Seminary School?"

Father Fredo smiled and proceeded to say, "I was only testing you to see if there was any fire in your soul." He continued, "You obviously have a strong sense of family, and it is this sense of famila that will not let you die. You have too much to live for and you are too ornery to give up." Father Fredo then surprised me. He told me,

"I'm Italian and my father's name was Corleone. Small blessings are the special parts of life that mean so much. They bring great joy. They are selfless acts of kindness – the times you help someone just because they need help, the jobs you do for the elderly and those who are less fortunate. It is the giving of one's self just for the giving and expecting nothing in return. John, I know you have given much during your life. Your name has been mentioned at services throughout the years. These small blessings give us a reason to live."

Father Fredo went on to say, "You are not going to die. I knew I was going to talk to you today even though I did not know you were here." Father Fredo then started to tell me about a dream he had last night. He said he had come from a very close family and that he was taught the value of helping others. His mother had told him that these small blessings will add up substantially over a person's lifetime and that there would be a time in his life that he would use these blessing to call on strength to get him through a crisis.

"My father came to me last night and told me about you. My Dad said that you were a good family man and that you needed to be reminded about the good you have done in your life. It was time for you to call on your special blessings to help give you the strength to live."

I lay in my hospital bed for the next few hours contemplating what Father Fredo had told me. I looked back on my actual family, thought of all the strength and support I had been given over the years, and how much I needed their support now. I thought about my career at the Health Department, and realized how much my co-workers were like family to me, and I discovered just how special our careers as public servants are.

So let me make you an offer you can't refuse.

Help others through random acts of kindness, treat people as if they are your family, and when it is your turn to face a crisis, you will be able to call on your special blessing to give you the strength to pull through. ☀

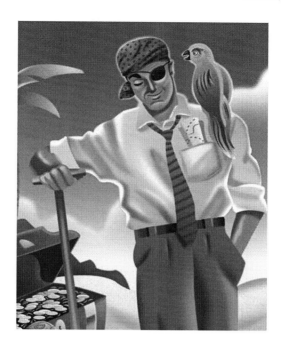

The Patch

By Mort Laitner

I had been lying in bed depressed for seven days. My son came into the room and as he dropped the mail on my lap said, "Dad, here's the mail, and there's an interesting package with no return address on it." Holding the manila envelope in my right hand, I looked through my right eye and observed it was postmarked Miami, Florida. My son was right; there was no return address. I remarked, "Travis, I wonder what's inside and who sent it."

I ripped it open, tearing the envelope into shreds. There it was, a rectangular box with a photo of a handsome young man wearing a pirate-style eye-patch. The box read CONVEX EYE PROTECTOR. A note was taped to the box. I silently read the note and shut my right eye as tears dripped down my face like an eye-dropper that misses its mark.

Travis asked, "Dad, are you okay?"

Eight days before the package arrived, I was at a party when electric sparks exploded inside my eyeball. My eye doctor repeatedly warned me that this would happen because my eyeballs were egg-shaped, and therefore, would likely detach and potentially cause blindness if not quickly patched. I knew that it was a detached retina having had this experience two years earlier in my other eye.

I immediately phoned my eye doctor, "Doc, my left eye is sparking. What should I do?"

The ophthalmologist responded, "Have someone drive you down to Bascom Palmer as soon as possible! I'll contact the on-call surgeon to be on standby to examine your eye and repair the detached retina, if necessary."

As I heard the doctor hang up, I thought about my last surgical experience. It wasn't so bad. The eye surgeon explained, "If the fluid leaks out of your eyeball, I'll have to fill it with air. And for the next ninety days, you'll spend your waking hours watching a TV which has been placed face-up on the floor with your head tilted in one position until the air pocket settles.

I prayed like I never prayed before. I used all of my mental powers. "Please Lord, no leakage." I knew if the fluid had leaked out my mental stability would collapse. I could not handle ninety days of TV torture. I would have ended up in a mental hospital. My prayers were answered when I awoke from the anesthesia. The first question I asked the nurse was, "Did the fluid leak out of my eye?" When I heard the nurse say no, I thanked G-d and fell back asleep.

Now, two years later, I was having a déjà-vu experience, same hospital, same condition, same surgery, and same prayers, but DIFFERENT RESULT.

I would have a buckle placed on my left eyeball. I already had one on my right, and if the buckles didn't coordinate with each other, I would have double vision. This time, my prayers were only partially answered. No leakage but no coordination. As each day passed, I grew more and more depressed. I asked myself, "Why me? How will I handle this?"

I thought about the people I knew who had disabilities. They all moved on with their lives. They embraced their disability with courage, fortitude and poise. They learned from it and were better because of it. I sat up in my bed and resolved, "No more pity, sadness nor tears. From this day on, I will embrace this challenge."

I opened the eye-patch box and stretched the black elastic band snugly over my head. It felt tight, but I no longer had double vision. This problem was solvable – no more headaches, no more seeing two of everything. I could now drive at night. I could read without closing my eye. But at what cost - the stares of children reacting to a one-eyed pirate? I decided I would salute them by giving them my best, "AAARGH!! Ahoy matey!" I would learn to love their facial reactions of bewilderment.

That original eye-patch is long gone, and I have bought many since then. But I still carry the anonymous tear-marked note in my wallet. I often pull it out as a reminder whenever I or a friend faces a crisis and read it out loud,

"EMBRACE THE CHALLENGE."

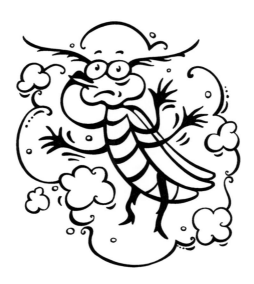

Metamorphosis

By Mort Laitner

One of the early lessons a public health attorney learns is that there are two types of environmental health inspectors. The type "X" inspector actively seeks out vermin with a Tony Montana attitude, "I'll bury those cock-a-roaches." While the Type "Y" inspector fails to see a Men in Black giant cockroach-like alien threatening the destruction of the planet.

Here is the story of two such inspectors Bill and Charlie.

I was accompanying these two gentlemen on separate days to learn about nursing home inspections.

On Tuesday, when Charlie and I entered the Miami Shoreline Nursing Home, we were greeted as royalty by the staff. It was an "unannounced" visit but the employees did not seem surprised. We were also greeted by the odor of human decomposition mixed with a heavy dose of deodorizer. Charlie appeared to have lost his sense of smell.

"Charlie, would you and your friend like some breakfast?"

"No!" Charlie exclaimed.

The staff looked bewildered.

"Well, how about a freshly brewed cup of java?"

"Not today, I'm training the health department lawyer."

Suddenly, their faces expressed an all-knowing look.

As we entered the kitchen, Charlie tightly held his clipboard professionally noting the name and address of the facility on his inspection sheet. At a quick pace, he rushed through the kitchen, not moving a pot or a pan. He carried no crack and crevice insecticide applicator spray to force the roaches out of hiding. I quizzed Charlie about his knowledge of roaches, "Charlie, are there different types of cockroaches?"

He answered, "I don't remember, but I think they're called German, Asian, Oriental and American."

Then I asked Charlie about the University of Florida study that I had recently read. Charlie was not familiar with the study that showed that cockroaches leave chemical trails in their feces, so other roaches follow the trails to discover food, water and where roaches are hiding.

What he did study was his inspection sheet. He acted like he had never seen one before. He never lifted his head to find a violation. His attitude was, "I do not live here, and who cares about the people who do."

Through all the bedrooms and bathrooms, Charlie did not find a single violation. Then we sat down in the administrator's office for Charlie to present his completed inspection form. We were again greeted like close family.

The administrator said, "Charlie, How are Grete, Gregor and Franz doing? Would you and the lawyer like some coffee?"

"We'll skip it today. Maybe next time. My family is doing fine. Thanks for asking." Charlie replied.

I was surprised that the administrator knew the name of Charlie's wife and kids.

Charlie commented, "You run a tip-top, ship-shape nursing home. Keep up the good work." This overly-friendly administrator smiled as he heard Charlie's findings.

As we left the home, I glanced at Charlie's work product, seeing no violations and an excellent rating. I felt dirty.

The next mornings, Bill, wearing his white ten-gallon cowboy hat, and I went on our unannounced inspection of Naranja Lakes Nursing Home. As we walked in the door, Bill greeted the staff with a loud ear-shaking, "Howdy!"

The metamorphic change on the staff's faces from smiles to frowns was as noticeable as a skunk at a lawn party. They remembered Bill from his last inspection. They recalled how hard they had to work to correct the health violations. The sheriff was back in town. Bill remembered how this administration did not want to pay for pest control services.

Bill bellowed, "These administrative folks are tighter than bark on a tree."

There was no offer of coffee or breakfast.

They wanted us to leave as quickly as we appeared.

Their hostile tone could be heard in their words, as Bill hunted down roaches like a hound dog.

"How can we help you?"

"Which parts of the home are you going to inspect?"

"Please wait here as we get the administrator."

They used all these dilatory tactics to slow us down so that the janitorial staff could get a jump start for some last-minute cleaning. Bill politely answered the questions, not stopping as we moved from room to room, smelling, eying, touching and spraying every nook and cranny of the home. Roaches jumped out of electrical sockets. He drew his white pen from his pocket and noted every violation from cockroaches to torn window screens.

Bill would often ask me while he recorded the violations: "Would you want your grandma to live here?"

I replied, "Absolutely not!"

"Then let's get this home in shape so someone else's grandma will live in a clean and safe home."

Bill knew roaches. He was aware that they can remain alive for a month without food, and that their lifespan was up to a year. Bill read the national study on factors that affect asthma in inner-city children which showed that cockroach allergens worsen asthma symptoms. Bill was acquainted the preventive measures to keep roaches out of nursing homes: food stored in sealed containers, using garbage cans with tight lids, frequently cleaning the kitchen and regular vacuuming. All of which were lacking at this nursing home.

As we left the home, I felt clean. I thanked Bill for mentoring me. In his best western accent he twanged, "Pardner, this ain't my first rodeo, so remember what you learned today." Then he rode off into the sunset in his white 1967 Mustang convertible.

Scratching my head, I thought about the differences between Bill and Charlie.

There are people, like Bill, who care. While others, like Charlie, have undergone a Kafkaesque transformation.

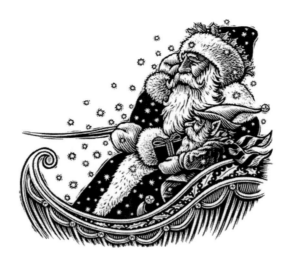

Santa's Helper

By Bobby Glass

As the clock hits 5:30, I am anxious to leave the office and start my trek home. I open the car door and inhale deeply. My little red car smells faintly of peppermint candy canes—thanks to my youngest son who decided to crush the candy and mush it into the back seat of my car. I climb in, and promise myself a steaming cup of hot chocolate, made with milk and topped with marshmallows. It is a bargain I make to get over my dread of the rush hour traffic that awaits me. To my amazement, there is almost none. I look over as I pass the Dolphin Outlet Mall and realize that my fellow commuters have all stopped on their way home to get in some extra shopping. I smile as I remember my recent trip to the mall on Black Friday. I never get tired of protecting my wife's "great deals" at 6 AM. I am pleased with our recent gift conquest for others and decide the minimal traffic is an early holiday gift from the universe. Making this realization then allows me to further enjoy my surroundings. I cannot help but grin when I see a smiling Santa gripping the Coke billboard to a red-berried, holly green wreath hanging on a white wooden door to ice-blue icicles drooping off of roofs. The spirit of Christmas is ultimate joy.

This is my favorite part of the year. Miami gets.. um.. cold, all of the stores decorate for the season, and holiday music plays all day on Love 94. As I continue my commute, I think about my holiday memories, the feel of ripping open a beautifully wrapped package early in the morning, the smells of a special dinner, the enjoyment of spending time with my family when I was younger, and now, how I am working to re-create these warm loving memories with my family. Stopping at a red light, I get excited when I think about my family traditions, watching our favorite holiday classics: It's a Wonderful Life and that Red Ryder BB gun special, A Christmas Story. I can't help but smile when I remember the line, "You'll shoot your eye out kid!" I remember how I wanted an "Official Red Ryder Carbine-Action Two-Hundred-Shot Range Model Air Rifle" as a child, and I chuckle when I think about how I turned out... a Safety Manager for over eight hundred people. For some reason (I am guessing it was the Burl Ives' Rudolph DVD I watched with the kids last night.. the one with the land of the reject toys), I think about Santa on the toy shop floor, overlooking the health and safety of the super fast toy producing elves. I notice the glow of the ruby light has now changed to an entrancing shade of emerald. My engine roars to life, and my holiday spirit leads me to back to all of the good fortune I have in my life.

I get excited as I increase my speed to merge into the turnpike traffic. I allow myself the liberty of imagining Santa in his sleigh, with gigantic reindeer attempting to do the same feat. Just how fast could a sleigh boasting nine veggie powered reindeer would fare against my 400 horse power engine?

I think Santa might have to stick to the city streets, because he would cause some serious accidents! I wonder how he stays safe with no seat belt, no doors to protect him from the elements, no helmet, and of course, an obscured view as he faces the backside of his reindeer. By now, I am almost home. My motorized sleigh knows the way through the warm winter streets.

Looking left out my window, I see station wagon laden with bags and bags of store-bought presents and an elderly man who looks like the guy in those Coke billboards: white beard, round face, and wire-rimmed glasses. He is talking on his cell phone. I observe his lips are pursed and can almost imagine him saying, "Ho, ho, ho!" I shake my head at my exuberant holiday spirit, and in a split second, my brain relayed something that instantaneously drained me of my holiday spirit. I had passively noticed his front passenger door was ajar, but when I was laughing to myself, my brain processed a danger that no family would ever want to think about. I looked further into the front of the car confirmed what my brain had already processed. Sitting next to the Santa-man was a small child, about three, with gleaming blond hair, and a face as beautiful as a tiny cherub. My alarm bells that sounded were screaming... door ajar. No child seat. DOOR AJAR. NO CHILD SEAT. NO SEATBELT! DO SOMETHING! I yell to the man and pointed at the girl, "You're door isn't closed!", but my timing was bad. The Look-a-like-Santa didn't hear me and drove away. I would be willing to bet he was probably thinking of a holiday to-do list. I accelerated and pull up along the side of his car. I check traffic in front of me, honk the horn, and signal to him that his passenger door isn't closed. The rosy color in his once happy cheeks drained when he too realized the danger his precious package was in. Faster than you can say, "Deck the Halls," he pulled off to the shoulder of the road.

As I pulled into my driveway, I was still thinking about the catastrophic events that could have happened. I got out of my car and walked into my house. I put on my green baseball cap to play catch with the kids. I love Florida in the winter. My youngest son ran to the door, took one look at me and said, "Daddy Elf". I laughed and picked him up. I glanced back at the mirror and realized I was wearing all green. My holiday spirit came back with a vengeance. I saved Christmas for one little girl. I had become, for a few seconds today, Santa's helper. I smiled again as I thought to myself, "No coal in my stocking this year!"

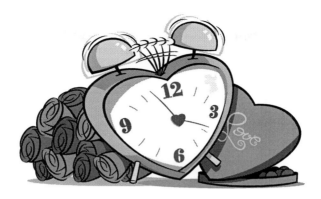

"Have I Told You Lately that I Love You" *Rod Stewart*

By John Holmes

The clock on the wall taunts me. I have a deadline to finish the performance evaluations for my staff. I have been reviewing them for days. I am proud that my staff has been successful in accomplishing every goal I have set for them in the last year.

My eyes wander to the calendar, and my brain freezes on the realization that today is Valentine's Day. Every year since we've been married, my wife wakes up to breakfast-in-bed and a gift on her breakfast tray.

Every married man's fear of forgetting Valentine's Day has just become my reality. The evaluations have preoccupied my mind causing me to forgot. Focusing on the evaluations will be impossible until I somehow decide what to do about my impending disaster. My spherical vision catches the picture of my wife and me taken on our wedding day; she seems to be looking right at me. My lower lip trembles when I realize her smile no longer appears happy and her Mona Lisa eyes are now following my every move in the office.

The little block in the lower right hand corner of my computer is flashing a notice that my administrator has emailed me an IMPORTANT message. I think to myself, "You do not know what important is until you experienced a man forgetting February 14!" I opened the email only to be faced with the evaluation deadline again. She states how important the evaluations are. I do not want to be disrespectful, but I am facing a crisis. I reply I am making good progress.

I think of a reasonable way my wife will understand that I forgot. I will tell her I am sorry and that we can celebrate this weekend combining her birthday. Yes, she will understand and forgive me because we are a team and we support each other in times like this. Who am I kidding! I am a dead man! What is worse is that I will be a dead man barely walking! Any man with half a brain knows you cannot reschedule an important date and try to combine two celebrations. Am I losing my mind?

My wife is going say, "Everything is alright, and do not worry about it. Just forget about this year and next year you will celebrate these dates properly." But I know she is still going to feel hurt.

I am losing time worrying about my love when I should be completing my evaluations. It is times like this that I wonder why I ever wanted to be a manager. My boss appears at my door to see how things are going. She sees that I am obviously stressed and asks if there is a problem. Reluctantly, I explain to her the situation I find myself in and how I do not know what to do.

She offers a suggestion to me, "Keep working on your evaluations for a couple more hours and take the rest of the day off so you can be with your wife. Immediately call a florist and have some expensive flowers delivered. Explain to the florist the dire situation you find yourself in and ask, beg if you need to, if they could expedite the delivery. In the card, tell her you will be home soon so you can properly celebrate Valentine's Day." I cannot believe my ears! My boss is helping me out of my problem. Thank God she understands.

I do everything my boss suggested and even offered to pay extra for the expedited delivery of the flowers after some embarrassing begging. One hour later, my wife calls to tell me of the surprise delivery and how she cannot wait for me to come home. A little while later, I arrive to a hero's welcome. It's like nothing happened. In the evening, we go out for an absolutely wonderful dinner. In the back of my mind, I keep thinking, "Why was my boss so understanding?"

We arrive back home and after a couple hugs and kisses, we go to bed and I fell asleep like there was never a problem.

The next morning, my wife fixes me a scrumptious breakfast and is as cheerful as I have ever seen her. I am about to finish eating and feel better about returning to the evaluations when my wife asks, "How much did you beg?" It is at this moment I realize that I had been setup by not only my wife, but my boss as well! She looks into my eyes and says, "Yes, I called your boss and told her everything. I also called the florist, told them the situation and to make you squirm a little." I laugh at loud and head to work.

I'm sitting at my desk polishing the evaluations when I glance at the clock and recognize that next Valentine's Day the breakfast, the gift, and my love will all be on my wife's tray. ☀

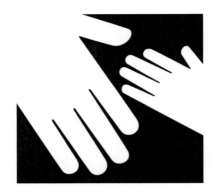

Grandfather's Hands

By Mort Laitner

My home is cold; ambient temperature 42 degrees.

I'm boiling a kettle of water for some Sanka.

As the coffee simmers I place my hands over the just-turned-off electric burner.

 I rub my hands together.

My hands and heart warm as I recall my grandfather.

His smiling image burned into my mind.

 I'm a four year old, living in a high rise in Astoria, Queens.

Winter chills the building.

My grandfather prepares his coffee on his gas range.

I observe his morning ritual: boil water, pour water into his striped blue and white porcelain cup, sip the black coffee, and then he returns to the stove to stretch his hands above the flame like a caveman standing near his campfire.

As my grandfather rubs his hands together, he stares at me as his face brighten with a life-is-good smile.

 A warm shelter, a job, a good cup of java and his grandson watching him start his day.

His heart and hands reach out to me with a hug and a kiss as he leaves for work. ☼

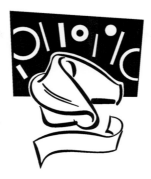

Ay Caramba
Las Cucarachas

By Mort Laitner

As I sat in the Chinese restaurant tasting the last drops of my Lobster Cantonese, the waiter dropped a plate of fortune cookies on the table. I grabbed one and ripped open its wrapping. Securing the cookie between my thumb and forefinger I squeezed. The cookie crumbled into four pieces exposing that sliver of white paper with its inked message. I reached over the plate and pulled the fortune toward my eyes:

THE SMART THING TO DO IS TO PREPARE FOR THE UNEXPECTED.

I thought, "Yeah, right, what a message; what wisdom scrawled on this note." Confucius modified the Boy Scout motto 2000 years before its birth.

As I left the restaurant, a cold fall night blanketed the city. A solitary street lamp's glare emitted enough light so that I could make out the red, yellow and orange maple leaves swirling to the ground.

As I hunted for my friend Neil's two-story Victorian, I was bundled in the uniform du jour, my woolen, navy pea coat and well-worn bell bottoms.

Tired from my adventures in lower Manhattan, I needed a hassle-free place to crash. Neil's invite sounded encouraging.

As I entered the old house, the smell of burning strawberry incense permeated my nostrils. I flicked on the hall lights observing a dozen cockroaches scurrying back under the floorboards.

I shrieked, "Ay caramba los cucarachas!"

Roaches were a serious hang-up.

"This can not be happening," I thought as Neil greeted me with a bear hug and loud, "How you doing buddy?"

"Not bad, how you doing?" I answered.

"You got any Raid?"

Neil replied, "Sorry bro, we ran out weeks ago. The cold weather will kill them in a few days."

I thought to myself, "I'm going to be here for only one night. The less time spent here, the better."

"Neil, lets go to an all-night diner for some coffee, my treat."

He muttered, "Sure Buddy, I got the munchies."

In the diner I pondered, how I was going to sleep in the infestation. The thought of bugs crawling on my lips, creeping into my ears, terrorized me.

I remembered the earwig episode of Night Gallery – little bugs tunneling through my brain causing excruciating pain.

On our return to the house, I turned on the black light in the living room, observing a bean bag chair, a day-glow psychedelic poster of Hendrix in a tie-dye shirt fingering his guitar and a worn-out, lumpy sofa, my bed.

Neil turned on his stereo, blasting the Stones, 'Gimme Shelter'.

I belted out the words, 'Gimme shelter from these nocturnal nightmares.'

I followed by yelling, 'Gimme shelter from these vermin.'

I scoured the rest of the room for black six-legged arthropods. Seeing none, I managed to fall asleep.

I dreamed of disease-carrying bugs, covering my body like a black velvet robe. Next, I was transported back to the diner's restroom where I studied myself in the wall mirror. 'No, no!' I cried as I saw my terrifying reflection. I shook my head frantically as roaches dropped from my hair like dandruff.

I woke shivering yet covered in sweat. I jumped up, throwing off my army-issue blanket and looked out the window. The diner's neon lights blinked,

OPEN 24 HOURS

I thought back to the fortune cookie,

"THE SMART THING TO DO IS TO PREPARE FOR THE UNEXPECTED."

I packed up my belongings, quietly shut the front door and spent the rest of the night sitting in the diner.

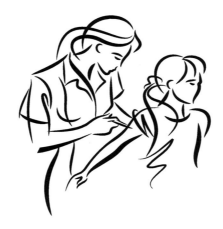

Health Department Barbie

By Morton Laitner

arbara Millicent Roberts, officially known as Barbie (that surprised me!) is fifty years old.

Barbie has been very career minded over the decades. She has been a teacher, doctor, nurse, dentist, actress, flight attendant (or stewardess depending on your generation) for three different airlines. Barbie has been in numerous military positions, United States president (our first -- don't tell Hillary), firefighter, babysitter, paleontologist (who would have thought), McDonald's cashier (created during the last recession) How many dolls do you think Big Mac bought? Barbie has been a cowgirl, chef, police officer, life guard (Baywatch of course), NASA astronaut, and a NASCAR driver (lots of fans)... She has worked more than 100 jobs.

But where is Health Department Barbie? With her resume, Barbie would make a great asset to our team!

According to designer Diane Von Furstenberg, "Barbie represents a confident and independent woman with an amazing ability to have fun while remaining glamorous." This sounds like all the female HD employees I know. I'm starting to get the picture, if you want Barbie in your profession you need to lobby Mattel.

Therefore, on behalf of all Health Department personnel

around the world, I am commencing the Health Department Barbie (HDB) campaign.

> We need your support.
> Write Mattel.
> Demand our doll.
> Promise you'll buy one.
> E-mail them your design for HD Barbie.
> Start a HDB petition drive.
> Create a HDB blog, web page or an e-zine.

I often hear HD employees state we don't get any respect (we are the Rodney Dangerfield's of professionals) out in the field or from our kids, or from our spouses or from our neighbors and friends.

Now is our opportunity to change all that.

Mattel will cave with our avalanche of requests.

And if they don't we'll just put little name tags on those doctors, nurses and dentists, even that paleontologist saying, **"Proud Health Department Employee."**

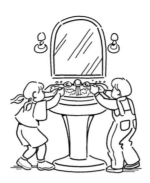

Wash Your Hands

By Amy Tejirian

Wash your hands
After you sneeze or cough
When you wash
It keeps all those nasty germs off

Wash your hands
Before you cook meat or any treat
Don't forget to wash
Before you eat

Wash your hands
After visiting the bathroom
You can wash
Using a soap with sweet smelling perfume

Wash your hands
When you come home
To properly wash
Scrub'em well and use lots of foam

Wash your hands
It's important to do
How long should you wash?
Sing Happy Birthday times two

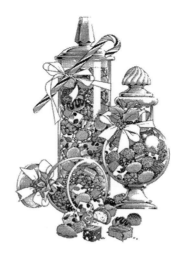

Add A Little Sugar

By Gerri LeClerc

Life without sugar
A bird without wing
A pool without water
A voice without sing

Life without sugar
A plant without flower
A class without teacher
A castle without tower

Life without sugar
Santa without beard
Life without sugar
Is just simply weird.

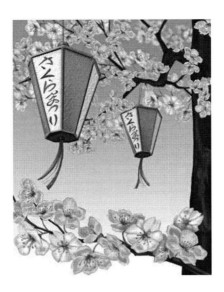

Healthy Haikus

By Tracie Dickerson and Amy Tejirian

Thin, fat, heart attack
Leafy greens and lean proteins
Keeps your body fit

Brush and floss your teeth
In the morning and evening
Avoid cavities

Babies cry hungry
Breast feeding is important
Formula for love

Walk, walk everywhere
Dance and sing and play today
Jump, jump, jump for joy

Plan for a big storm
Water, flashlight, batteries
Keep sane in hurricanes

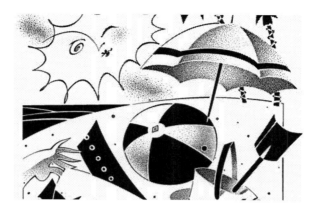

The Sun

By Maryann Bean

When I go out in the sun
Sunscreen is number one

Aloe kote goes on my nose
Then I start from head to toes

May Kay SPF 15 goes on my face
It comes in an oil-free base

Bain de Soleil on the arm and on the chest
Then I continue with the rest

On my back goes SPF number 8
Hurry up it is getting late

Down on my legs to my feet
SPF you cannot beat

When we were young having fun
We stayed out too long in the sun

Now skin cancer has come to stay
So I protect myself today

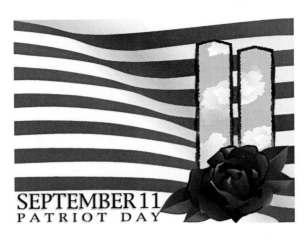

SEPTEMBER 11
PATRIOT DAY

Terrorism 2002

By Maryann Bean

Who would have thought back in 1992
The next disaster would be bigger than Andrew

Hurricanes, floods and tornados were our threat
Now terrorism is far bigger, you can bet

Where and what the next act will be
Will involve both you and me

Are you ready to stand up and serve
Or will the next act throw you a curve

Many things you will need to know
So to the next training session you better go

You may be exempt from serving for some reason
But remember that terrorism has no season

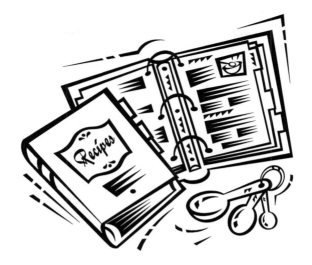

Tamar's Tasty Pate

By Tamar Scheinberg

Lentil Pate - Mocked Chopped Liver

3 TBS olive oil
1 medium onion, coarsely chopped
3 garlic cloves, coarsely chopped
1/2 tsp. dried oregano
1/4 tsp. dried thyme
1 cup tasted walnuts
1 cup cooked lentils
1/4 tsp. Dijon mustard
1/3 tsp. fresh lemon juice
2 hard cooked eggs
Salt & pepper to taste

Heat olive oil in a small skillet on medium heat. Sauté onions and garlic about 2 minutes - till soft, not brown, then let cool.

In a food processor with metal blade, add all ingredients and the sautéed onions and garlic, then process until smooth. Season to taste and chill.

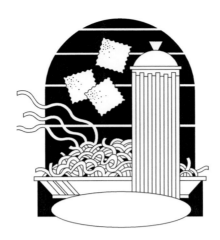

Pasta Chuta

By Hasmig Tejirian

Sauce Blanche

Add 5 cups of milk to a sauce pan. Heat milk on medium until bubbles barely start to form before boiling - do not boil the milk.

In a separate small bowl mix 5 tablespoons of white flour with 5 tablespoon of soft butter (room temperature).

Whisk vigorously the flour/butter mixture into the hot milk The milk will eventually start to boil and thicken.

Remove the milk from the heat.

Add a pinch of salt, black pepper, and any other spice you want (like a pinch of nutmeg or herb de provence).

Adding the Cheese

Add 12oz of shredded cheese (preferably a 3 cheese blend - if not then only mozzarella will do) to the sauce blanche.

Noodles

Cook 1 package of egg noodles according to the directions on the package (keep it aldente, because we will complete the cooking in the oven).

Add the noodles to the cheesy sauce blanche mixture.

The final steps

Butter the 9x13" pyrex dish.

Pour in the completed mixture.

Bake at 400 degrees for 15 minutes

Sprinkle some cheese on top and back for another 10 minutes (or less until slightly Golden).

Bon Apetit!

Variations

You can use 4cups of milk (instead of 5) with similar adjustments to the butter and flour, but please remember to take away 1/5 of the noodles as well.

You can also use whole wheat flour but make sure it is a rounded tablespoon for each cup of milk.

You can also use whole wheat noodles.

Hasmig Tejirian is a Kindergarden teacher in Los Angeles, California.

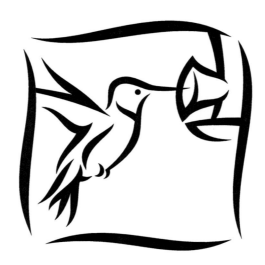

The Institute:
A Risk Taking Story[1]

By: Tracie Dickerson
Story Related by: Lillian Rivera

Looking out my office window, I smiled as I saw a monk parakeet feeding her chick. I thought about my career with the Health Department and the projects that I have focused in on. One of these endeavors was the Florida Public Health Institute. I thought back to the morning I discovered a study entitled, "The Potential of America's Public Health Institutes."[2] Delving deeper into the report, I found that California, Michigan and Louisiana were already operating successful enterprises. I remember thinking, "Wow! This project would be beneficial to all Floridians. How will I get this off the ground?" In this moment of clarity, I decided that this venture would be part of my legacy.

I contacted the two institutes to learn how they were created.

1 An institute is a permanent organizational body created for a certain purpose. Often it is a research organization (research institution) created to do research on specific topics. An institute can also be a professional body. In some countries institutes can be part of a university or other institution of higher education, either as a group of departments or an autonomous educational institution without a classic full university status such as a University Institute.
2 The genesis of the National Network of Public Health Institutes was a 1999 conducted by the Michigan Public Health Institute entitled "The Potential of America's Public Health Institutes". The study reviewed the nine state public institutes (PHIs) in existence and argued that their emergence amounted to a national movement for innovation and efficiency in the US public health system

My ears resonated when the Director of the Michigan Institute said, "We have a multi-million dollar budget and commensurate staff." I knew this project would entail extensive commitment of time, but when I thought about the benefits to the community, I knew the journey would be worth it.

A Senior Leadership meeting was convened to brainstorm the idea. Everyone except our lawyer was enthusiastic about the project.

As lawyers often do, she said, "Lillian, I hate to burst your bubble BUT I do not think there is any legislative authorization for a Health Department to create a Public Health Institute." My face must have shown my disappointment because the lawyer then said, "You know, there might be a way to do this, but I need to do some research."

The next day, the attorney called me, she said "The Legislature recognizes the importance of meeting the needs of public health professionals and that is one of the goals of any institute, so it may fly. The Legislature emphasizes that there is a unique partnership which exists between the state and counties in meeting the public health needs. We could team up with some universities and incorporate the institute."

I replied, "Let's do a risk/benefit analysis. I am going to contact my bosses in Tallahassee and see if this idea ruffles their feathers."

The lawyer said, "The risks are minimal, especially if we started the process by going to the County Commission for an ordinance to authorize the creation of an Institute."

I said to her, "I've stuck out my neck many times before and have had my hand slapped, on a few occasions, but as moral dilemmas go, this is a no-brainer. It would cost me a few bucks, but I have always known to be a leader you must be a risk taker."

We found organizations and universities willing to partner with the fledgling institute. Then we filed our corporate documents and obtained the recommended county ordinance. Faculty members at the University of Miami Miller School of Medicine and at the Florida International University Stempel School of Public Health agreed to serve on our board of directors. It was slow going at first. There were board meetings and small projects such as the Public Health History Tour[3], but nothing close to the caliber that I envisioned. I

3 A tour of where the Tequesta Indians inhabited on the mouth of the Miami River, the cemetery where bodies were buried from the

did not want to watch this project fade away. I was at wits end. We had worked so hard to get to this point, but where were the sponsors? How could we make this project grow? When would we have our millions?

While we were contemplating, Tallahassee voiced its opinion on our creation. The Agency attorney came to see me and said, "Well, we got our analysis regarding our Institute from Tallahassee. What do you want to hear first, the good news or the bad?"

I responded, "I always like hearing the good news first."

The lawyer said, "County Health Departments can actively participate in not-for-profit corporations. This means we can partner with UM and FIU in the Public Health Institute."

I snapped, "What's the bad news?"

She said me, "They said County Health Departments cannot operate or create a not-for-profit corporation."

I replied, "Well, we're not operating it. We are only going to be a member of board." I looked my attorney in the eye and said, "I've got some great news." "Dr. Earl Fox, from University of Miami, is going to take the institute to the next level. He is going to make permanent headquarters in Lantana and he is going to get the grants to make this institute, the FPHI[4] viable[5]."

A year later, at a Senior Leader meeting, I announced, "Great News, The Institute6[6] received operation funding ($1.25 million) from the National Network of Public Health Institutes/Robert Wood Johnson Foundation and the Quantum Foundation." I then told my staff, "The Institute has created four Centers for Health Workforce development, Preventive and Primary Care, Education Research and Training, and Bioterrorism and Health System Readiness."

---

epidemics of cholera, yellow fever, and Spanish flu, the Alamo (Miami's City Hospital which opened in 1918), and the Orange Bowl and its use as a quarantine station and refugee holding area, and Al Capone's home where he died of syphilis. While riding on the bus, participants were lectured by a local historian and during breaks, listened to classic health related songs such as Keith's "98.6" and "Good Lovin'" by the Young Rascals.

4 In 2006, the Public Health Institute was renamed as the Florida Public Health Institute.

5 Today, FPHI has formed partnerships with the Town of Lantana, Nova Southeastern University, University of Miami, Florida Department of Health, A.G. Holley Hospital, Palm Beach and Miami-Dade County Health Departments, Florida International University, University of South Florida School of Public Health, and Florida Atlantic University, among others. In 2008, FPHI merged with the Florida Public Health Foundation, located in Jacksonville, Florida.

6 It is our vision that FPHI will evolve into an Institute with multiple governmental and private funding sources with connections to all academic public health institutions in Florida. These affiliations will bring additional intellectual capital to enhance health care services and an improved health system fabric throughout the state and nationally. FPHI has already begun to form the necessary strategic partnerships to address education, research and policy issues. To date, FPHI has organized a two week "Masters Course in Public Health" with the cooperative assistance of seven universities from across the state, developed a county/state Public Health Nursing Workforce project, been chosen as lead Institute for a CDC national preparedness modeling project, coordinated a local partnership to present a business focused bio-preparedness health summit in November 2007 and is currently planning a 2008 health summit highlighting national and international water technologies and safety issues.

"I just learned," I said, "that we are being invited to participate in the institutes two-week Masters Course in Public Health which has the assistance of seven universities across the state. Further, our nurses can participate in the institute's Public Health Nursing Workforce project." I was elated when I announced "that the Institute was chosen as lead for a CDC national preparedness modeling project, coordinated a local partnership to present a business focused bio-preparedness health summit in November 2007. Looking at my Environmental engineer, I advised him "the Institute was planning a health summit highlighting national and international water technologies."

As the monk parakeet flew off to find more food for its young, I smiled and considered the announcements I made at the Senior Leadership meeting that morning. I grasped my thought for the day, "A good idea, with a great team, and a little risk taking sometimes pays off big."

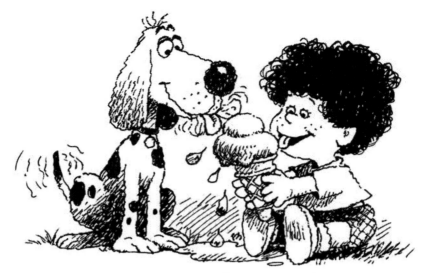

Sharing Our Best Practices

By Tracie Dickerson

The editors of Healthy Stories are proud to announce a new section of our book entitled, "Sharing Best Practices" we are requesting our readers to contribute their best practices for possible publication.

Many of us learned about sharing from having watched Sesame Street. Ellen DeGeneres taught Elmo to share his head phones. Cookie Monster and Hairy Monster learned about sharing a bicycle from Kermit. Parents can buy their kids the Sesame Street DVD; "Learning to Share" where Elmo discovers that sharing with friends makes playtime twice as much fun. The DVD contains a song entitled "Sharing" and a claim that it helps make growing up a lot more fun, which for many of us those growing up pains literally hurt.

We at the Miami-Dade County Health Department and our supporters have taken the sharing message to heart. Here is one of our ideas that we're sharing:

Statewide Quarantine Facility Library

1. Start the process by creating a lending library—save on gas to library or bookstore, recycle your unwanted forms of entertainment and cost of purchase of books, magazines, movies or music. Save paper—save a tree-- e-mail request to friends and employees.

2. Ask your staff to donate (share) their books, DVDs, CDs and board and video games.

3. The policy is for every item you take out of the library you must substitute another item.

4. Collect a few hundred books and the other entertainment items.

5. Change the name of the lending library to "name of health department quarantine facility library" and get volunteer staff to agree to transport the whole collection to a quarantine facility during an event.

6. Share idea with other public health leaders from other regions of state to have numerous quarantine libraries for use in major event.

7. Save the tax payers the burden of purchasing entertainment items for the quarantined.

8. Remember sharing is fun. ☼

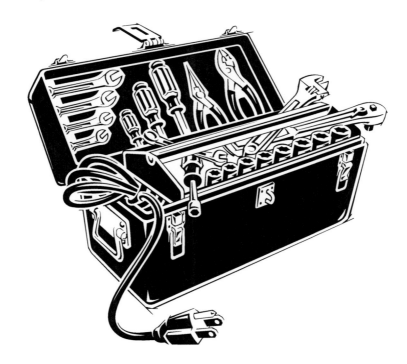

The Matrix

By Mort Laitner

It was the best of times, it was the worst of times, and it was the epoch of the matrix (apologies to Charles Dickens for modifying the firs sentence of his classic, "A Tale of Two Cities."). As we move from good to not so good times, we re encouraged to modify our behavior and, in other words, "change."

In the opinion of the authors in their #1 book on change, "Who Moved My Cheese," the Spenser Johnson's message is simple: When your cheese disappears you have two choices: (1) wait to be bailed out (usually preserved for banks and sometimes done by the legislature for governmental agencies) or (2) put on our sneakers and start searching for new cheese.

If your included to put on the sneakers, inside the shoe, you will find a road map designed like a matrix, a number two pencil and instructions. While lacing your sneakers, read the instructions:

PROACTIVELY IS YOUR GREATEST TOOL

1. Do not sit on your hands as others decide your economic fate.

2. Cut your costs with your own knife

3. Use this cost-reduction matrix as your scalpel.

4. Take the pencil and fill in the portion entitled Supplies and Equipment.

5. Gather Data. How many cell phones, Blackberries, copiers do you possess? Look at your inventory, your employees' phone bills. Let them know via email that you are monitoring their phone usage.

6. As you fill in the matrix, take time to focus in on your strategic priorities.

7. Determine the difference between luxuries and necessities.

8. Seek the cooperation and recommendations of your team.

9. Make the hard decisions and explain those decisions to your staff.

10. Realize as political leaders mandate reductions in expenditures, you have already cut a layer of fat from your beloved bureaucracy.

11. Remember the most important column on the matrix is the "actual savings to the agency" area. This area can only be completed with documented, empirical data.

12. Review your matrix every two weeks in front of your team. Praise the money savers. Be prepared to reevaluate your cost savings measures.

13. Celebrate your successes as you watch the savings grow.

14. Be creative and share your successes.

Thanks for carefully reading these instructions. Now that your sneakers are on, and you are holding your pencil, get moving, collect data, search out waste, cut luxuries, and remember to celebrate your successes.

WINNER OF THE
2008 BEST STORY COMPETITION

A Survivor's Love Story

By John Holmes,
Environmental Health Director,
Putnam County Health Department

Dedicated to Marianne

I walked into the Key West Women Infants and Children (WIC) office with tears running down my cheeks. "Marianne is not coming," I told my friend. I was trying to explain while holding back the sobs which were tearing at my heart. "I just talked to her on the phone; she decided not to come. We planned this for almost two years. Now it is completely over. She asked me to ship her belongings back to her. The worst part is she has asked I not contact her anymore!"

Marianne is the love of my life. We met at Rochester Institute of Technology in New York where we lived in the same campus building. My wife left me shortly after school started. Marianne was dealing with a failing marriage of her own. It all started innocently. I would see her outside reading or just relaxing under a tree after work. We would talk casually about school and our past. Marianne is Dutch. She lived in the United States for almost 30 years. We talked about places we had both visited. Time with Marianne made the grueling class schedule almost bearable. We walked from campus housing to the health center following streets and a shortcut through the woods directly behind the campus.

Almost imperceptibly, we moved emotionally closer. Neither of us knew what was happening. We started holding hands and would say goodbye with a hug. Marianne was invited to an awards banquet; she asked me to accompany her. It was a cool misty evening outside the Eastman House in Rochester that night. We sat through the ceremony which was followed by a dinner with music and dancing. We were enjoying the evening and decided to step outside for some fresh air. The mist had changed to a light drizzle so we decided to sit near a grape arbor -- an overhead trellis on which grape vines grow. We sat next to each other to stay warm. Mellowed on wine we found ourselves in a romantic atmosphere. I turned to Marianne, looking into her kaleidoscope eyes and said, "I love you." She looked at me and replied, "ik houd van jou," which is Dutch for I love you. My heart was beating in my throat and my head was pounding. I then said to Marianne, "I want us to be together forever." Marianne replied, "I have felt the same way for quite awhile."

Our love continued to grow and soon we decided to get married. There were many difficulties to overcome, but it was inevitable we would be together.

I was in a state of shock as I was sitting in the chair in the WIC office trembling with a chill. My mind was disconnected from my body. My thoughts were only of Marianne. Now what would I do? My friend tried to console me, but I was too devastated to comprehend what had just happened. I contacted my supervisor and explained that I was not feeling well and needed to go home for the rest of the day.

At home, I felt empty. I sat in disbelief at my situation. Slowly I collected Marianne's personal belongings for shipment. It took several days to complete what should have taken a few hours. Each item held a memory. I was packing and shipping my love and dreams. It was the most difficult task I had ever done. As my dreams where being weighed and tagged for shipment, I decided that I was not going to fall to pieces. I was going to lose myself in my work. I was going to work so hard that I would not have time to think about Marianne. I did not know that my future would bring the most difficult time of my life. In my pain of losing Marianne, I could not have comprehended there would be a time in my near future when I would have a brush with the Angel of Death.

Work became my obsession. Double-duty workloads did not give me the peace I craved. The harder I tried, the more troubled I became. It did not make sense -- the way Marianne ended our plans. I just could not accept it. I thought that if I could work myself to exhaustion, I could at least escape her when I slept. Sleep was fitful.

I created a business so I would have additional work to fill my nights and weekends and give me extra money to help solve my growing financial crisis.

My financial crisis began when I was in my forties with a family and had injured my back. I decided that the only way I would be able to support my family was to earn a college degree. I had over-estimated what my market value would be when I graduated. This led me to believe that I would be able to repay my massive student loans. My debt load upon graduation was beyond my ability to pay. I hoped the additional income from the side business would solve my problems. First, it would distract me from the painful end of my relationship with Marianne and, second, it would help pay-off my debts. After several months, it was obvious that my debt coupled with the high cost of living in The Keys was unmanageable. I decided to take the most humiliating solution to my financial problems and I filed for bankruptcy. I had become a bankrupt, broken-hearted loser. I guessed by now that maybe Marianne was right. She somehow sensed that I was really a loser and I was beginning to believe it.

Bankruptcy eliminated much of my debt, but not all. I still had to pay back my student loans, yet it did help some. I needed to either get a raise or a promotion. I realized that without one or the other my career would soon be over and I would need to seek other employment.

My opportunity came quickly when my supervisor decided to retire unexpectedly. I was the next senior inspector in the office and I had been through several staff turnovers already. Now was my time to be rewarded for my loyalty and hard work. I felt a buoyancy that helped push my problems to the background. I looked forward to going to work again. I almost smiled again, something I had not done in a long time. I secretly thought to myself: just wait Marianne; you will see that I am not a loser. The day of the interview proved again that, yes, I am a loser. I was now a bankrupt, rejected loser.

I was devastated at this new loss. I realized I had only one avenue to follow -- leave the Keys. I decided to transfer to another health department.

My search did not take long. I was offered a job in a small rural county in the northeast part of the state. I would be promoted and the cost of living was substantially less. This was the best news I had in many years. I accepted the job and made plans to transfer. I finished all my open cases and left for my new life. I had no idea where I would live or what it would cost. All I cared about was a new beginning.

When I arrived, the first place I went was to a motel to make plans to stay for several weeks until I could find someplace to live. It did not take long. One of my co-workers knew a person who had a place to rent. I checked it out and took it. I finally had a new home.

Time passed quickly and I became a part of the team immediately. I needed some retraining because there are many differences in Environmental Health between the Keys and where I was now working. I learned quickly and settled down to live my new life. Marianne was always with me. I thought about her everyday. Time had dulled the pain, but the memories were still vivid. I did not talk to anyone about her, but I think that sometimes I seemed distracted with something.

A year and a half later, I was driving between inspections with a colleague. I told her I was having a terrible pain in the middle of my back and I needed to stop to walk it off. We stopped and it went away after quite some time. I had an annual physical scheduled in a couple days and made a mental note to tell my doctor about it.

I took the day off for my physical and was there 15 minutes early (I operate on Lombardy time). The receptionist took my information and put me in the exam room where I waited for the doctor. When he arrived, we had the usual discussion and I told him about the pain in my back. He ran an EKG and after examining the results, told me I had experienced a heart attack and needed to have a stress test immediately. I told him that I did not have time for one right now, but I would have one when I returned from a trip later that week. I had planned to help drive my friend's car to Phoenix and fly back. I was only going to be gone a few days. The doctor said he would not recommend the trip and said it was imperative that I get the test. I relented and agreed to have the test the next day. Again I arrived 15 minutes early, ready to put this all behind me. Besides, I was okay and the doctor was just being overly cautious.

The test went quickly. It was a thallium treadmill test. I had a little trouble completing the treadmill part, but I was just out of shape. The cardiologist returned with the results and told me it indicated a major blockage. He said I should have an angiogram immediately. I told him thanks, but no thanks; I had a trip to go on and would have it done when I returned. He told me that I may not make it back, that the heart attack I experienced would probably be my only warning. The next one would in all likelihood be major if not fatal. Again, I agreed to have the test and it was scheduled for the next day. I completed the test and the results showed that I needed open heart surgery as soon as possible. I was taken from the exam area to an ambulance where I was transferred to a hospital in Jacksonville for surgery the next day. Marianne really had broken my heart.

I awoke with a pipe in my throat! I could not swallow and was in a panic. I wanted the pipe out right now. The nurse told me I needed to calm down and it would be removed as soon as possible. They needed to leave the pipe there so I would continue to breathe in case there was a problem. Eventually, the pipe was removed and I was able to calm down. I was returned to intensive care for recovery. When the doctors decided I was doing fine, they would return me to the recovery area and finally to my room. I was heavily sedated and not able to comprehend anything, but after several days in intensive care, I figured there was something wrong. I asked questions and realized that all was not right. There was trouble in the operating room, my heart did not start up right away and my abdominal organs were not working properly. My kidneys were not working. In other words, I was slowly dying and nobody knew what to do. I wished I could say goodbye to Marianne. I wanted her to lie next to me so I could hold her as I slipped away. I wanted my last words to be, "I love you." Later that night I awoke in a morphine induced state of disillusionment and self-pity. I turned to buzz the on duty nurse and as I watched the door, suddenly, I envisioned a faceless-dark-hooded figure. I remember wondering if the grim reaper had come to harvest my soul.

After five days, I still was not recovering well enough, so they decided to do a complete CAT scan of my chest and abdomen. It was a cold January night when they took me for the test. I was shivering uncontrollably. They rolled me into the scan room and took so many scans I should have glowed in the dark. I was returned to my room to wait for the results the next day. When my doctor came to my room, he was not alone. He brought an oncologist. He said they had found a large tumor near my kidney and it would need to be removed as soon as I was well enough to withstand the trauma. The doctor said that the tumor was resting on a large artery causing a condition called Deep Vein Thrombosis (DVT) which is essentially an accumulation of clots in my leg. This could lead to any number of serious, if not fatal, complications. The one positive fact in all this gloom was that the tumor was encapsulated which essentially gave me more time, but I could not wait forever.

For whatever reason, I started to recover shortly after the CAT scans and was returned to my room where I remained for an additional 10 days. I continued to improve in most respects, but was having trouble walking. The nurse had me up several times a day walking the halls and finally I was well enough to go home to heal from my heart surgery.

I was recovering at home and trying not to worry about the upcoming surgery. My friend Diane was staying with me as a live-in nurse. She went through the ringer with me. I could not sleep right; would not eat. Nothing tasted like it was worth eating. About three weeks after I was home, I fell ill again and returned to the hospital. It seemed my kidneys were failing again. I do not know what happened, only that I eventually returned home to continue my recovery and try to gain enough strength to have the next surgery. I wondered if Marianne realized just how much I loved her and how badly she broke my heart.

About two months after the bypass surgery I returned to the hospital to have the cancer removed. The tumor was so large it had to be removed from the front. While the surgery was excessively invasive, there were no complications. I started to recover almost immediately and within ten days returned home. I continued my slow recovery. Diane needed to leave to take care of some family business, so a co-worker at the health department said I could stay with him and his wife until I could care for myself. That amounted to three weeks. I was now in my home able to get around, but my recovery was not progressing well. I did not have the spirit to go on. I wondered if it was all worth it. I just didn't care. I had been through so many heartaches, so many disappointments; now I was a complete physical mess! Why was I being beat-down so bad? I could not find a reason to continue or to try to get well.

I took a road trip to visit my parents who lived about 50 miles away. I was not sure I could drive that far, but decided to try. I arrived at my parent's home exhausted from the drive. I went inside, had a drink of water and went to the spare bedroom to take a nap. When I awoke, mom had cooked a meal and was waiting for me. We talked and I told them about how lucky I was to be alive. After the meal, my mother brought me a letter from "an old friend of mine" that had arrived a couple of days earlier. I was stunned to find it was from Marianne! She wrote that she was trying to find me. She wanted to apologize for the way our relationship ended. Marianne enclosed all her contact information so I could find her if I wanted.

The anger rose in my throat. It was blocked by my memories of our love. I wanted to yell at her and hold her tight at the same time. I realized I was stomping around in my parent's home and decided to sit in an effort to calm down. I read the letter repeatedly trying to decipher what she might really be saying. I placed the letter in my pocket until I returned home. I read, re-read, and re-re-read and still could not get it out of my head that there was more-than-what-met-the-eye. That same night I replied to her letter in which I told her about moving and the promotion. I wrote that I was happy with my life. I had a new friend who was French and cared for me. She stayed with me during my health issues. I went on and on. I wanted Marianne to know that I did not need her anymore. I even signed the letter "sincerely." The one time in my life when it meant the most, my anger overruled my heart. I sent the letter and that was that.

Two days later I received a phone call. The Caller-ID showed it was Marianne! I let it ring several times and reluctantly answered it. I heard her voice and all my anger melted and turned to tears. I knew that I still loved her as if nothing had ever happened. Marianne apologized for what had happened. She reminded me that her mother was gravely ill at the time she was to come to me and passed away shortly after that. I could hear her softly crying on the phone when she said she never stopped loving me. She expressed that she always believed one day we would be together. As she continued, I realized she never had abandoned me. Marianne had entrusted me with her heart. She never took it back. I asked her to forgive me for doubting her love. We must have talked for hours. When we realized that we had talked long enough, I asked what she wanted to do now. Could we meet somehow? She told me she had just gone through cancer surgery herself and could not travel very far. We decided to meet in Valdosta, Georgia.

A couple of weeks later we met. To see the two of us together one would have been shocked. I could not get out of my truck by myself. Marianne had lost so much weight that I might have missed her on the street. We were about as pathetic as two people could be. Marianne helped me out of my truck. We hugged, we kissed and we knew we would be together for the rest of our lives.

We met in Valdosta a couple more times. My recovery was slowly improving. We were making our plans for our future together. On our last trip we visited San Mateo, Florida, and looked at a house to purchase. Marianne thought it was ugly until I told her how I envisioned our home. When we went inside she found the house welcoming. I knew we would live there soon. We went back to the motel and decided to make an offer. We moved in three months later.

Although my health problems were not over, I knew everything would be fine. Shortly before we moved into our home, I developed a condition that required a cervical fusion. I had surgery without any problems and felt as if I could have jumped off the operating table and gone home. Marianne was at my side the whole time, and that was all that mattered. Marianne was taking a break from her life to recover also. She was gaining weight and smiling again. I was glad she was able to recover with me.

Guess what? Three months later I had surgery again; I had my gallbladder removed! Fifteen months: four surgeries, two mended hearts.

Now as I walk into the WIC office, tears of joy run down my face as I tell Diane the rest of the story. Marianne and I are happily married. I have been promoted to senior management. Marianne has become an American citizen. Both of us have fully recovered and are cancer free for over five years.

WE AND OUR LOVE HAVE SURVIVED.

Historia de Amor
de un Sobreviviente

Dedicado a Marianne

Yo entraba a la Oficina de Mujeres, Bebés y Niños (WIC) de Key West con lágrimas corriendo sobre mis mejillas "Marianne no regresa," le dije a mi amigo. Lo decía mientras trataba de aguantar mi llanto que estaba haciendo pedazos mi corazón. "Yo acabo de hablar con ella por teléfono, y ella ha decidido no regresar. Nosotros hemos planeado esto por casi dos años. Ahora está completamente terminado. Ella me ha pedido que le envíe sus pertenencias. ¡La peor parte es que ella ha pedido que yo no la contacte más!"

Marianne es el amor de mi vida. Nos conocimos en el Instituto de Tecnología de Rochester en Nueva York donde vivimos en la misma residencia de estudiantes del Instituto. Mi esposa me dejó poco después de que las clases comenzaron. Marianne también estaba pasando por un fracaso matrimonial. Todo comenzó inocentemente. Yo la veía a ella leyendo afuera o simplemente relajándose bajo un árbol después del trabajo. Hablamos casualmente sobre la escuela y nuestro pasado. Marianne es Holandesa. Ella ha vivido en los Estados Unidos por casi 30 años. Hablamos de lugares que los dos habíamos visitado. El tiempo con Marianne hizo ese inaguantable horario de clases soportable. Caminamos de las residencias de estudiante al centro de salud siguiendo calles y un atajo a través del bosque directamente detrás del las propiedades universitarias.

Casi imperceptiblemente, nos acercamos emocionalmente. Ninguno de los dos sabíamos lo que estaba pasando. Comenzamos agarrándonos las manos y a decirnos adiós con un abrazo. Marianne fue invitada a un banquete de premios; y me pidió que la acompañara. Era una fría nebulosa noche fuera del Eastman House en Rochester. Nosotros atendimos la ceremonia la cual continuaba con una cena con música y baile. Estábamos disfrutando la noche y decidimos ir afuera para tomar un poco de aire fresco. La neblina había cambiado a una suave llovizna por lo que decidimos sentarnos cerca de una pérgola de uvas – un armazón elevado por encima de nuestras cabezas sobre la cual crecen los viñedos. Nos sentamos uno al lado del otro para mantenernos calientes. Suavizados por el vino nos encontramos en una romántica atmósfera. Yo me dirigí a Marianne mirando hacia sus kaleidoscopios ojos y le dije, "Te quiero." Ella me miró a mi y respondió, "ik houd van jou," que en Holandés significa te quiero. Mi corazón estaba latiendo en mi garganta y mi cabeza estaba palpitando, Luego le dije a Marianne, "Yo quiero que estemos juntos para siempre." Marianne respondió, "Yo he sentido lo mismo desde hace cierto tiempo."

Nuestro amor continuó creciendo y pronto decidimos casarnos. Había muchas dificultades que superar, pero era inevitable que estaríamos juntos.

Yo estaba en un estado de shock mientras estaba sentado en una silla en la oficina de WIC temblando de la ansiedad. Mi mente estaba desconectada de mi cuerpo. Mis pensamientos eran todos sobre Marianne. ¿Ahora que haría yo? Mi amigo trataba de consolarme, pero yo estaba muy devastado para comprender lo que acababa de pasar. Yo contacté a mi supervisor y le expliqué que no me sentía bien y que necesitaba irme a la casa por el resto del día.

En la casa, me sentía vacío. Me senté con escepticismo ante mi situación. Poco a poco, recogí las pertenencias de Marianne para enviárselas. Tomó varios días completar lo que ha debido tomar solo unas horas. Cada cosa traía recuerdos. Estaba empacando y enviando mi amor y sueños. Era la tarea más difícil que alguna vez yo había hecho. Mientras mis sueños estaban siendo pesados y etiquetados para envió, yo decidí que no me iba a hacer pedazos. Yo me iba a perder en mi trabajo. Yo iba a trabajar tan duro que no tendría tiempo de pensar en Marianne. Yo no sabía que el futuro me traería los momentos más difíciles de mi vida. En mi dolor por perder a Marianne, no podía haber comprendido, que mi futuro cercano traería tiempos en los que me iba a encontrar con el Ángel de la Muerte. El trabajo se convirtió en mi obsesión. Jornadas de trabajo doble no me dieron la paz que yo deseaba. Lo más duro que yo trataba, lo más perturbado que me ponía. No tenía sentido - la manera en la que Marianne terminó nuestros planes. Yo simplemente no lo podía aceptar. Pensé que si yo podría trabajar hasta estar exhausto, podría al menos escapar de ella mientras dormía. El dormir era disturbado. Yo creé un negocio para tener trabajo adicional a fin de llenar mis noches y fines de semana y darme dinero extra para ayudar a resolver mi creciente crisis financiera.

Mi crisis financiera comenzó cuando yo estaba en mis cuarenta con una familia y me había lastimado mi espalda. Yo decidí que la única manera de que yo era capaz de sostener a mi familia era adquiriendo un título universitario. Yo había sobreestimado lo que mi valor de mercado sería cuando me graduara. Esto me llevó a pensar que yo iba a ser capaz de pagar mis masivas deudas estudiantiles. El monto de mi deuda al graduarme era mayor que mi habilidad de pagarla. Yo esperé que el ingreso adicional de mi negocio particular resolviera mis problemas. Primero, me distraería a mí del doloroso final de mi relación con Marianne y, segundo, me ayudaría a pagar mis deudas. Después de varios meses, era obvio que mi deuda conjugada con los altos costos de vivir en Key West era no manejable. Decidí tomar la más humillante solución a mis problemas financieros y peticioné la declaración de bancarrota. Yo me había convertido en un perdedor en bancarrota y con el corazón roto. Creía para el momento que quizás Marianne estaba correcta. Ella de alguna manera sintió que yo era en realidad un perdedor y estaba comenzando a creerlo.

La declaración de bancarrota eliminaba bastante de mi deuda, pero no toda. Yo todavía debía pagar las deudas de mis préstamos estudiantiles, aunque ayudaba en algo. Necesitaba obtener un aumento de sueldo o una promoción. Yo me di cuenta que sin uno el otro pronto mi carrera habría terminado y yo hubiese tenido que buscar otro empleo.

Mi oportunidad vino rápido cuando mi supervisor decidió retirarse repentinamente. Yo era el siguiente inspector con más experiencia y había pasado por varios cambios de personal. Ahora era el momento de ser premiado por mi lealtad y duro trabajo. Sentí un optimismo que ayudó a empujar mis problemas hacia atrás. Estaba entusiasmado con volver a trabajar otra vez. Yo casi volví a sonreír otra vez, algo que no había hecho en mucho tiempo. Yo pensé: tan solo espera Marianne; ya verás que no soy un perdedor. El día de la entrevista probó otra vez que, sí, yo era un perdedor.

Yo estaba devastado por esta nueva derrota. Me di cuenta que solo tenía una avenida que tomar – dejar los Keys. Decidí solicitar la transferencia a otro departamento de salud.

Mi búsqueda no tomó mucho tiempo. Me ofrecieron trabajo en un condado rural pequeño en la parte nordeste del estado. Yo sería promovido y los costos de vida eran sustancialmente menores. Esta era la mejor noticia que yo había tenido en muchos años. Yo acepté el trabajo e hice los planes de transferir. Terminé todos mis casos abiertos y comencé mi nueva vida. No tenía idea dónde viviría ni cuánto me constaría. Todo lo que me importaba era un nuevo comenzar.

Cuando llegué, al primer sitio que fui fue a un motel a hacer planes para quedarme por unas semanas mientras encontraba un sitio donde vivir. No tomó mucho tiempo. Uno de mis compañeros de trabajo sabía de una persona que tenía un sitio para arrendar. Lo vi y lo tomé. Finalmente tenía un nuevo hogar.

El tiempo pasó rápido y yo formé parte del equipo de trabajo inmediatamente. Necesitaba cierto reentrenamiento ya que hay muchas diferencias con relación a salud ambiental entre los Keys y donde estaba ahora trabajando. Yo aprendí rápido y me establecí a vivir mi nueva vida. Marianne estaba siempre conmigo. Pensé en ella todos los días. El tiempo había ensombrecido el dolor, pero los recuerdos estaban todavía vivos. Yo no hablé con persona alguna sobre ella, pero pienso que a veces parecía distraído con algo.

Un año y medio después, yo estaba manejando entre inspecciones con una colega. Yo le dije que tenía un terrible dolor en el medio de mi espalda y necesitaba parar para aliviarlo. Paramos y se me fue después de cierto tiempo. Yo tenía programado un examen físico anual en un par de días e hice una nota mental a fin de comentarle a mi doctor sobre ello.

Me tomé el día libre para el examen físico y estaba allí 15 minutos antes de la cita (yo opero sobre tiempo Lombardy). La recepcionista tomó mi información y me puso en el cuarto de examen donde esperé al doctor. Cuando él llegó tuvimos la discusión usual y le dije sobre mi dolor en la espalda. Él realizó un EKG y después de examinar los resultados me dijo que yo había experimentado un ataque al corazón y necesitaba tener un examen de stress inmediatamente. Yo le dije que yo no tenía tiempo para uno en ese momento, pero que yo me lo haría cuando regresara de un viaje luego esa semana. Yo había planeado ayudar a manejar el carro de mi amigo a Phoenix y volar de regreso y solo iba a estar fuera unos días. El doctor dijo que él no recomendaba el viaje y que era imperativo que yo me hiciera el examen. Yo concedí y acorde hacerme el examen al día siguiente. Otra vez, llegué 15 minutos antes, listo para poner todo esto detrás de mí. Además, yo estaba bien y el doctor solo quería ser muy cuidadoso.

El examen fue rápido. Era un examen de estera de thallium. Tuve un poco de problema completando la parte de la estera, pero solo estaba fuera de forma. El cardiólogo retornó con los resultados y me dijo que indicaban un bloqueo mayor. Me dijo que yo debía tener un angiograma inmediatamente. Yo le dije gracias, pero no gracias; yo tenía que ir a un viaje y me lo haría cuando regresara. Me dijo que podría no regresar, que el ataque al corazón que experimenté podría ser mi única advertencia. El próximo sería más grave sino fatal. Otra vez, acordé hacerme el examen y fue programado para el siguiente día. Completé el examen y los resultados mostraron que yo necesitaba una cirugía de corazón abierto lo antes posible. Yo fui llevado del área de examen a una ambulancia donde fui transferido a un hospital en Jacksonville para la cirugía al día siguiente. Marianne de verdad me había roto el corazón.

¡Me desperté con un tubo en mi garganta! No podía tragar y estaba en un estado de pánico. Yo quería que me quitaran el tubo en ese momento. La enfermera me dijo que me tenía que calmar y que iba a ser removido lo antes posible. Ellos necesitaban dejar el tubo allí a fin de que yo continuara respirando en caso de algún problema. Eventualmente, el tubo fue removido y yo pude calmarme. Fui retornado al área de cuidado intensivo para recuperación. Cuando los doctores consideraron que yo estaba bien, me regresaron al área de recuperación y luego a mi cuarto. Estaba bastante sedado y no era capaz de comprender nada, pero después de varios días en cuidados intensivos, me imaginé que algo andaba mal. Pregunté y me di cuenta que no todo estaba bien. Hubo problemas en el cuarto de operación, mi corazón no comenzó a funcionar allí mismo y mis órganos abdominales no estaban trabajando apropiadamente. Mis riñones no estaban trabajando. En otras palabras, yo estaba muriéndome poco a poco y nadie sabia que hacer. Yo deseé poderle decir adiós a Marianne. Yo quería que ella estuviera al lado de mí de manera que pudiera agarrarla mientras me iba. Yo quería que mis últimas palabras fueran, "te quiero." Luego esa noche me desperté en un estado inducido por morfina de desilusión y compasión propia. Me viré a murmurarle a la enfermera de turno y mientras miraba a la puerta, repentinamente, visualicé a una figura oscura con capucha sin cara. Yo recuerdo haberme preguntado si el nefasto colector había venido a recoger mi alma.

Después de cinco días, yo todavía no estaba recuperándome lo suficiente, por lo que decidieron realizar un examen de CAT de mi pecho y abdomen. Era una fría noche de enero cuando me realizaron el examen. Yo estaba temblando incontrolablemente. Me llevaron al cuarto de examen y me hicieron tantos exámenes que yo podría haber brillado en la oscuridad. Fui regresado a mi cuarto a fin de esperar por el resultado de los exámenes al día siguiente. Cuando el doctor vino a mi cuarto él no estaba solo. Él trajo a un oncólogo. Dijo que habían encontrado un tumor muy grande cerca de mi riñón y que debía ser removido tan pronto yo estuviera lo suficientemente bien para soportar el trauma. El doctor dijo que el tumor estaba sobre una arteria mayor causando una condición llamada Trombosis de Vena Profunda (DVT), lo cual era esencialmente una acumulación de coágulos en mi pierna. Esto podría conducir a un sin número de serias, sino fatales, complicaciones. El único hecho positivo en toda esta miseria era que el tumor estaba encapsulado, lo cual esencialmente me daba más tiempo pero no podía esperar para siempre.

Por la razón que fuera, me comencé a recuperar poco después de los exámenes de CAT y fui regresado a mi cuarto donde permanecí por unos 10 días adicionales. Me continué mejorando en casi todos los respectos pero tenía problemas caminando. La enfermera me paraba varias veces al día a fin de caminar en los pasillos y finalmente estaba en condiciones de irme a mi casa a recuperarme de mi cirugía de corazón.

Me estaba recuperando en la casa y tratando de no preocuparme por mi siguiente cirugía. Mi amiga Diane se estaba quedando conmigo como enfermera a tiempo completo. Ella vivió la agonía conmigo. No podía dormir bien; no podía comer. Nada sabía como que valía la pena comérselo. Alrededor de tres semanas después de estar de vuelta a casa, me sentí mal otra vez y regresé al hospital. Parecía que mis riñones estaban fallando otra vez. Yo no sé que pasó, solo que eventualmente regresé a casa para continuar mi recuperación y tratar de ganar fuerzas para mi siguiente cirugía. Me pregunté si Marianne se imaginaba tan solo cuanto la amaba y lo mal que rompió mi corazón.

Alrededor de dos meses después de la cirugía de corazón regresé al hospital para que me removieran el cáncer. El tumor era tan grande que tuvo que ser removido por el frente. A pesar de que la cirugía fue bastante invasiva no hubo complicaciones. Yo comencé a recuperarme casi inmediatamente y al cabo de 10 días regresé a la casa. Continué una recuperación lenta. Diane necesitó irse a fin de atender un asunto de negocio familiar, así que un compañero de trabajo del departamento de salud dijo que me podía quedar con él y su esposa hasta que yo pudiera valerme por mí mismo. Ello tomó alrededor de tres semanas. Estaba ahora en mi casa pudiendo hacer cosas, pero mi recuperación no estaba progresando bien. No tenía el espíritu de seguir adelante. Me preguntaba si de verdad valía la pena todo esto. Simplemente ni me importaba. Yo había pasado por tantas tristezas y desilusiones; ahora yo era un completo desastre físico. ¿Por qué había sido golpeado tan mal? No podía encontrar razón alguna para continuar o para tratar de mejorarme.

Fui por carretera a ver a mis padres quienes vivían a 50 millas de distancia. No estaba seguro si yo podía manejar tan lejos pero decidí tratar. Llegué a la casa de mis padres exhausto del viaje. Entré, tomé un poco de agua y fui al cuarto auxiliar para tomar una siesta. Cuando me desperté, mi mamá había cocinado algo de comer y me estaba esperando. Hablamos y les dije sobre la suerte que tenía de estar vivo. Después de comer, mi mamá me trajo una carta de "una vieja amiga" que había recibido dos días antes. ¡Estaba sorprendido de ver que era de Marianne! Ella escribió que estaba tratando de encontrarme. Ella quería disculparse por la forma que nuestra relación había terminado. Marianne anexó toda su información de contacto de manera que yo la pudiera localizarla si quería.

La rabia creció en mi garganta. Estaba bloqueada por los recuerdos de nuestro amor. Quería gritarle y abrazarla al mismo tiempo. Me di cuenta que estaba zapateando alrededor en casa de mis padres y decidí sentarme en un esfuerzo por calmarme. Yo leí la carta varias veces tratando de descifrar lo que ella quería decir. Guardé la carta en mi bolsillo hasta que regresé a casa. La leí, la re-leí y la re-re-leí y todavía no pude quitar de mi cabeza que había algo más. Esa misma noche le contesté su carta en la cual le escribí sobre mi mudanza y la promoción. Le escribí que estaba contento con mi vida. Que tenía una amiga francesa que me cuidó. Que se quedó conmigo durante mis problemas de salud. Continué y continué. Quería que Marianne supiera que no la necesitaba más. Hasta firmé la carta diciendo "sinceramente". Lo que me importaba más en un momento de mi vida, mi rabia lo anuló. Envié la carta y eso fue todo.

Dos días después recibí una llamada telefónica. ¡La identificación de llamada indicó que era Marianne! Lo dejé sonar varia veces y sin ganas lo respondí. Oí su voz y toda mi rabia se esfumó y se convirtió en lágrimas. Supe que todavía la amaba como si nada hubiese pasado. Marianne se disculpó por lo que había pasado. Ella me recordó que su madre estaba gravemente enferma cuando debía regresar a mí y murió poco después. Yo podía oírla a ella llorando suavemente a través del teléfono cuando ella dijo que nunca había dejado de amarme. Ella expresó que siempre creyó que algún día estaríamos juntos otra vez. Mientras continuaba, me di cuenta que nunca me había abandonado. Marianne me había entregado su corazón. Nunca se lo llevó. Le pedí que me perdonara por dudar de su amor. Debimos haber hablado por horas. Cuando nos dimos cuenta de que habíamos hablado lo suficiente, le pregunté que qué quería hacer ahora. ¿Nos podríamos encontrar de alguna manera? Me dijo que ella acababa de tener una cirugía de cáncer y que no podía viajar muy lejos. Decidimos encontrarnos en Valdosta, Georgia.

Un par de semanas después nos encontramos. Vernos el uno al otro juntos fue sorprendente. Yo no me podía bajarme de mi camión por mi mismo. Marianne había perdido tanto peso que podría haberla no conocido en la calle. Los dos estábamos bien patéticos. Marianne me ayudó a salir de mi carro. Nos abrazamos, nos besamos y nos dimos cuenta que íbamos a estar juntos para el resto de nuestras vidas. Nos encontramos en Valdosta dos veces más. Mi recuperación estaba poco a poco mejorando. Estábamos haciendo nuestros planes para nuestro futuro juntos. En nuestro último viaje visitamos San Mateo, Florida, y miramos una casa para comprar. Marianne pensó que era horrible hasta que le dije como yo imaginaba nuestro hogar.

Cuando entramos le pareció la casa acogedora. Supe que pronto viviríamos en ella. Regresamos al motel y decidimos hacer una oferta. Nos mudamos en tres meses.

A pesar de que mis problemas de salud no estaban terminados, pensé que todo iba a estar bien. Poco después de que nos mudamos a nuestra nueva casa, desarrollé una condición que requirió una fusión cervical. Me sometí a una cirugía sin problema alguno y me sentí que pude haber saltado de la cama de operaciones y haberme ido a casa. Marianne estaba a mi lado todo el tiempo, y eso era todo lo que me importaba. Marianne se estaba tomando un tiempo para ella misma a fin de recuperarse también. Ella estaba recuperando peso y sonriendo también. Yo estaba contento de que ella pudiera recuperarse conmigo.

¿Adivina qué? Tres meses después tuve cirugía otra vez; ¡Me quitaron la vesícula! Quince meses: Cuatro cirugías, dos reparaciones de corazón.

Ahora cuando entro a la oficina de WIC, lágrimas de regocijo corren sobre mis mejillas mientras le cuento a Diane el resto de la historia. Marianne y yo estamos felizmente casados. He sido promovido a la posición de Manager. Marianne adquirió la ciudadanía Americana. Ambos estamos totalmente recuperados y hemos estado libres de cáncer por más de cinco años.

NOSOTROS Y NUESTRO AMOR HEMOS SOBREVIVIDO

WINNER OF THE
2008 BEST STORY COMPETITION

A Survivor's Love Story
Creole Translation

By John Holmes,
Environmental Health Director,
Putnam County Health Department

Se pou Marianne li dedikase istwa sa a

Mwen tap mache antre nan biwo pwogram (pou fanm ti bebe ak ti moun) WIC ki nan Key West la, dlo tap koule nan je mwen, krye tap roule desann sou figi mwen "Marianne ale li pap tounen ankò mwen te di zanmi mwen yo.

Mwen tap eseye esplike yo pandan ke mwen tap kenbe yon okèt ak tout krye ki tap fann kè mwen. Mwen fèk pale ak li nan telefòn li deside pou li pa tounen ankò. Nou te travay sou sa pandan plis ke de zan. Kounye a ke tout bagay fini nèt ant nou li te mande mwen pou mwen xpedye bali tout sa ke li te posede bò isit la.

Sa kite pi rèd li mande mwen pou mwen pa chèche wè li ak pale ak li ankò ditou.

Marianne se yon fi ke mwen renmen tankou de je nan tèt mwen. Nou te fè konesans nan yon kote yo rele Rochester Institute of Technology nan New-York, nou tou le de te ap viv nan menm bilding ki gen apatman nan inivèsite a.poumounn rete.

Madanm mwen te kite mwen lè lekòl la te fèk kòmanse, Marianne pou kont pa li te ap goumen ak yon maryaj ki tap bal tèt chaje.

Tout bagay te kòmanse senpleman san okenn move lide oswa kalkil mwen te rankontre ak li lè li tap li liv li deyò anba yon pye bwa lè sa li te ap relax apre li te fini travay. Nou te pale kè pòpòz de lekòl nou, de lavi nou avan ke nou te rankontre. Marianne sòti nan peyi Laoland. Li te ap viv nan peyi lèzetazini depi plis ke trant lane. Nou te pale de kote ke nou tou le de te al vizite avan ke nou te rankontre. Ti moman ke mwen te pase ak Marianne yo te fè ke mwen te kapab sipote orè kraze zo klas nan lekòl la.

Nou mache ansanb depi apatman pou etidyan nan inivèsite yo jouk nan sant santé a, nou te pase nan rakousi epi nou te pase nan rak bwa yo ki te dèyè inivesite a. San nou pa te rann nou kont nou te vini bon zanmi, kòkòt ak Figaro. Nou tou le de pa te rann nou kont de sa ki tap pase nou. Nou te komanse kenbe men epi lè nou te ap di orevwa nou te konnen anbrase. Yo te envite Marianne nan yon fèt pou bay moun glwa ak konpliman bèl akolad, li te mande mwen pou mwen ale avèk li. Se te yon aswè ki te fè fre epi te gen bouya nan nwit sa a nan Rochester nan Eastman House. Nou te chita nan seremoni a apre sa yo te sèvi manje epi apre manje moun te komanse ap danse. Nou te kontan jan fèt la te ye nan swa sa a epi nou te deside pou nou soti deyò pou ale pran yon ti frechè. Yon ti farinaj lapli te ranplase ti bouya a, akòz de sa nou te deside al chita anba yon tonèl rezen. Fèy branch rezen yo te kouvri tonèl la. Nou te chita yonn bòkote lòt pou nou te kenbe kò nou cho. Kòm si ti diven nou te bwè a te fè nou gri nou te sou bò fè bèl romans. Mwen vire gade Marianne je mwen te fixe nan je pa li ki tap voye limyè nan tout kote tankou koukouy epi mwen te di li ke mwen te renmen li. Li te gade mwen epi li te reponn mwen" ik houd van jou" ki vle di mwen renmen ou nan lang moun peyi laoland pale. Kè mwen tap bat, goj mwen ak tèt mwen tap bat tankou tanbou kata lè sa a. Mwen di Marianne "Mwen vle pou nou toujou ansanb pou tout rès vi nou "Marianne te reponn mwen " mwen santi menm bagay ak ou depi kèk tan."

Lanmou nou te kontinye ap grandi epi byen vit nou te deside pou nou marye. Te gen anpil pwoblèm pou rezoud pou ke maryaj la te kapab fèt , men nou te konnen ke anyen pa tap kapab anpeche nou fè vi nou ansanb.

Mwen te tankou yon moun ki pral endispoze lè ke mwen te chita nan chèz nan biwo pwogram WIC la, mwen tap tranble ak frison, bonnanj lespri mwen te kite kò mwen. Tout lide mwen te sou Marianne sèlman. Ki sa mwen dwe fè kounye a ? Zanmi mwen yo te eseye konsole mwen, men mwen te pran yon two gwo chòk pou mwen te konprann sa ki te fèk rive mwen a. Mwen rele bòs sipèvizè travay mwen epi mwen te esplike li ke mwen pa te santi mwen byen, ke mwen te bezwen ale lakay mwen pou rès jounen a.

Lè mwen te rive lakay mwen mwen te santi mwen vid. Mwen te chita san ke mwen pa te vle kwè ke sa ki tap pase mwen a se te laverite. Men trennen mwen pran tan, men mwen ranmase zafè Marianne yo pou mwen voye yo ale bali. Li pran mwen anpil jou pou mwen te fè travay sila a ke mwen te kapab fè nan yon ti kadè de tan.

Chak zafè Marianne ke mwen tap ranmase te fè mwen sonje li. Mwen te ap ranmase ak xpedye lanmou mwen ak rèv mwen. Se te travay pi difisil ke mwen te janmen fè. Pandan yo tap peze epi mete etikèt sou rèv mwen yo pou voye yo ale, mwen te deside ke mwen pa tap pèdi kontwòl lavi mwen. Mwen tap pral mete tout kouraj mwen nan travay mwen. Mwen ta pral travay di tèlman ke mwen pa tap pral gen tan pou mwen sonje Marianne. Mwen pa te konnen ke jou ki tap vini nan lavi mwen yo ta pral jou ki tap pi difisil nan tout lavi mwen. Nan doulè ke mwen te santi de se ke mwen te pèdi Marianne mwen pa te kapab konprann ke te gen jou ki tap vini ke mwen tap pral troke kònn mwen al lanmò.

Travay mwen te tounen tout vi mwen, menm lè ke mwen te travay de fwa plis kantite lè travay ke mwen te dwe fè, mwen pa te janm jwen lapè mwen tap chèche a. Plis mwen te eseye travay pi di mwens mwen te jwen lapè tèt mwen. Jan ke Marianne te fini plan nou yo ak maryaj nou a pa te fè sans ditou. Mwen pa te kapab aksepte sa ki te pase a. Mwen te kwè ke si mwen te touye tèt mwen anba travay jouk mwèl mwen te fè mwen mal mwen ta kapab chape anba pwoblèm yo lè ke lè a te vini pou mwen domi. Men mwen pa te kapab domi anpè. Mwen te fè yon biznis pou mwen te kapab genyen plis travay pou okipe mwen lè li aswè ak pandan wikend samdi dimanch, anplis tou pou mwen te fè lajan anplis pou ede mwen rezoud gwo pwoblèm lajan ki tap trakase mwen.

Gwo pwoblèm manke lajan pou peye bil mwen, te komanse lè ke mwen te genyen karant lane sou tèt mwen ak yon fanmi pou mwen okipe pandan ke mwen te fraktire do mwen. Mwen te deside ke sèl jan mwen te kapab kontinye okipe fanmi mwen se te pou mwen al etidye nan inivèsite pou mwen genyen yon diplòm ak yon metye. Mwen te konprann ke lè mwen te pran diplòm la mwen tap kapab fè yon pakèt lajan epi tou ke mwen tap kapab peye pakèt dèt mwen te fè pou mwen te kapab al etidye nan inivèsite a. Lè mwen te fini lekòl ak jwen diplòm mwen, lajan ke mwen te dwe a te plis ke sa mwen te kapab peye. Mwen te espere ke lajan ke mwen ta pral fè nan biznis mwen te fè apre travay mwen a tap pral ede mwen rezoud pwoblem mwen. Tou dabò li tap distrè mwen pou retire lide mwen sou jan zafè ak Marianne la te fini nan tèt chaje a, epi tou li tap ede mwen peye dèt mwen.

Apre plizyè mwa tout moun te kapab wè ke mwen pa te kapab vini about ak pwoblèm lajan anba gwo dèt mwen yo epi tou lavi chè nan zòn yo rele Keys nan Florida.

Mwen deside pou mwen pran solisyon ki pi desann eskanp figi moun lè yo gen pwoblem lajan, mwen te deside pou mwen krye fayit sa yo rele icit bankrupcy. Mwen te vini yon moun an fayit, yon bon aryen ki te pèdi tout bagay menm lanmou moun ke li te renmem ak tout kè li.

Mwen sipoze ke Marianne te gen rezon nan yon sans li te santi ke mwen se te yon moun kip pa tap remèt anyen epi mwen te komanse kwè ke se vre ke mwen te konsa tout bon vre.

Paske mwen te deklare ke mwen te an fayit mwen te kwè ke tout dèt mwen yo te fini, men se pate tout ki te fini vrèman mwen te oblije kontinye peye dèt mwen te fè pou peye lekòl ak viv pandan ke mwen te lekòl la. Men fayit la te ede mwen plizoumwens. Mwen te bezwen oswa ke yo ban mwen yon ogmantasyon nan travay mwen oswa ke yo te ban mwen yon promosyon nan travay la ki tap vle di plis lajan. Mwen te realize ke san yonn oswa lòt karyè mwen kote ke mwen te ye a ta pral fini nan yon ti tan epi ke mwen te ap oblije al chèche lòt travay.

Opòtinite pou plis lajan te vini byen vit lè sipèvizè mwen a te deside pou li pran retrèt li san atann. Nan biwo mwen a se te mwen menm ki te enspektè ki te pi wo grade apre sipèvizè a. Mwen te wè anpil chanjman nan travay la, kounye a se te tou pa mwen pou yo te rekonpanse mwen de se ke mwen te rete tout tan sa alòs ke lòt moun te ale anplis tou poupou yo te rekonpanse mwen pou tout kouraj mwen te mete nan kraze kò mwen nan travay di tou tan sa yo. Mwen te santi san mwen te ap mache pi vit, sa te ede mwen mete pwoblem mwen yo dèyè tèt mwen pou moman sa a. Nan epòk sa a mwen te rekòmanse gen kè kontan lè mwen ta pral ale nan travay la. Mwen te ap souri yon bagay ke mwen pa te fè depi lontan lontan. Mwen te di tèt mwen an sekrè tann pou ou wè Marianne, ou va wè ke mwen se pa yon moun ki fini, ki pap remèt anyen. Jou mwen te ale nan reinyon pou yo te mande mwen keksyon pou wè si mwen te kapab vini yon sipèvisè sa pa te mache ditou. Yon lòt prèv ke mwen se te yon moun ki fini tout bon vre, ki te an fayit nan tout jan, ke lasosyete te rejte.

Paske mwen te pèdi promosyon nan travay la se te yon lòt malè ki te ravaje mwen, Mwen te realize ke sèl bagay ki te rete pou mwen te fè se te kite kote mwen tap viv la nan Keys nan Florida. Mwen te deside pou mwen mande transfè mwen nan yon lòt depatman lasante nan yon lòt kote.

Li pa te pran mwen anpil tan pou mwen te jwen yon lòt travay. Mwen te jwen yon travay nan yon ti konte nan zòn riral nan pati nòtès nan leta Florida. Yo te ban mwen yon promosyon epi lavi laba a tap koute mwen chè. Se te pi bon nouvèl ke mwen te jwenn depi plizyè lane.Mwen te asepte travay la epi mwen te fè plan mwen pou mwen transfere. Mwen te fini tout travay ke mwen te kòmanse sa te vle di fèmen tout ka ke mwen te komanse epi ale nan lavi tou nèf ki tap tann mwen. Mwen pa te gen okenn lide de kote ke mwen ta pral viv la oswa de kantite lajan mwen tap bezwen pou mwen viv nan zòn la. Tout sa ki te enpòtan pou mwen se te ke mwen tap pral rekòmanse ak lavi mwen. Lè mwen rive nan kote riral la premye kote mwen ale se te nan yon motèl kote mwen te fè plan pou mwen rete pandan plizyè semen jouktan mwen ta va jwen yon kay kote pou mwen rete. Li pa te pran anpil tan pou mwen te jwen yon kote, yon moun ki te ap travay nan menm kote ak mwen te konnen yon moun ki te genyen yon kote pou lwe. Mwen te tcheke kote a epi mwen te lwe li. Anfin mwen te genyen yon kote nèf pou mwen te viv.

Tan a te pase byen vit epi mwen te fè pati ekip travay la tou swit. Mwen te bezwen pou yo ban mwen antrenman pou mwen te kapab fè travay la paske travay sante anviwònman nan Key West ak kote ke mwen te ap travay la nan zòn riral la pa te menm bagay. Mwen te aprann byen vit tout sa mwen te bezwen konnen pou mwen te kapab fè travay la epi mwen ranje kò mwen pou mwen viv lavi tout nèf mwen te rekòmanse ap viv la. Lide mwen te toujou sou Marianne, mwen te ap sonje li chak jou ki te ap pase. Tan ki te pase yo te kalme doulè a, men souvni Marianne yo te frèch nan tèt mwen. Mwen pa te pale de li ak pyès moun, men gen de fwa mwen te sanble ak yon moun ki te gen tèt li ki pa te la.

Yon lane edmi te finn pase mwen te ap kondwi pou mwen al fè enspeksyon yo ak yon lòt anplwaye travay mwen. Mwen di li ke

mwen te genyen yon doulè anraje nan rèl do mwen epi ke mwen te
bezwen rete yon ti moman pou pran yon souf. Nou rete epi doulè a
pase apre yon bon moman. Nan kèk jou mwen te gen pou mwen ale
lakay doktè mwen pou li te tcheke mwen tankou tout moun dwe fè
chak lane, epi mwen di tèt mwen pou mwen sonje di doktè a zafè
doulè ki te pase mwen a.

Mwen te pran yon jou konje pou mwen te ale lakay doktè a, mwen
te rive nan klinik la kenz minit avan lè randevou mwen a (Mwen se
yon moun ki mache sou lè Lombardy). Resepsyonis nan klinik la te
pran enfòmasyon mwen epi li te mete mwen nan yon sal egzamen
kote mwen te rete tann doktè a. Lè doktè a te rive sou mwen nou
te pale sou sa doktè ak patyan konnen di nan konsiltasyon, epi tou
mwen te di doktè a ke mwen te konn gen doulè nan rèl do mwen.
Doktè a fè yon egzamen elektrokadyogram epi apre ke li finn gade
tès la li di mwen ke mwen te fè yon atak kote ke kè mwen te sispan
bat pandan yon moman. Li di mwen ke mwen te bezwen fè yon tès
tou swit pou wè kijan ke kè mwen travay lè yo mete estrès sou li.
Mwen te di doktè a ke mwen pa te genyen tan pou mwen fè yon
tès kounye a men ke mwen va fè tès la lè mwen tounen sòt nan
yon vwayaj ke mwen te ap pral fè nan semen ki ap vini a. Mwen te
genyen yon pwojè pou mwen te kondwi machin yon zanmi mwen pou
ale nan kote yo rele Phoenix epi pou mwen tounen nan avyon. Mwen
tap ale sèlman pou dezoutwajou. Doktè a te di mwen ke li dekonseye
mwen fè vwayaj la epi ke li trè ekzijib pou mwen te fè tès la tou swit.
Mwen te fè ranka, men mwen te dakò pou mwen fè tès la jou anapre
a. Nan jou an apre a mwen te rive tou kenz minit pi bonè tou pare ke
mwen te ye pou mwen fini ak koze tès kè sa a. Anplis mwen te pote
mwen trèbyen epi doktè a tap ekzajere nan pran twòp prekosyon.

Tès la te fèt byen vit. Se te yon tès sou yon machin kote yo mete
moun kouri epi gade kijan kè li bat. Mwen te gen difikilte pou mwen
te fini tès la, men se pa te anyen paske mwen te konnen ke mwen pa
te an plen fòm fizik. Doktè espesyalist kè a retounen ak rezilta yo
epi li di mwen ke mwen te genyen yon blokaj nan venn kè mwen. Li
di mwen ke mwen te bezwen fè yon tès ki rele anjyogram tout swit.
Mwen te di li mèsi bokou doktè mwen regrèt men mwen pap ka fè
tès la paske mwen gen yon vwayaj pou mwen al fè. Mwen di doktè
kè a ke mwen va fè tès la lè mwen retounen. Doktè a di mwen ke
mwen ka pa janm retounen sòt nan vwayaj sa a paske nan eta ke kè

mwen te ye a atak kè mwen te fè a ak doulè mwen te santi a se te sèl avètisman ke kè a te ban mwen. Prochen fwa ke mwen ta va fè yon lòt atak kè li ap yon gwo atak epi li kapab touye mwen. Mwen vinn dakò pou mwen fè tès la epi yo ban mwen randevou pou jou anapre a.

Mwen fè tès la epi rezilta yo te montre ke mwen te bezwen yon operasyon kote doktè yo ta pral louvri kè mwen pou yo koupe kote ki te bloke a kidonk pi bonè se te granm maten.Yo te fèm soti nan sal egzamen a nan yon anbilans ki te mennen mwen nan lopital Jacksonville pou operasyon kè a ki te pou fèt nan jou an apre a. Marianne te vreman kraze kè mwen

Lè mwen te leve mwen te genyen yon tiyo nan gòj mwen. Mwen te ap bat kò mwen, mwen te vle pou yo retire tiyo a menm moman a. Enfimyè a te di mwen pou mwen kalme mwen paske yo ta va retire tiyo a lè ke yo te kapab. Yo te oblije kite tiyo a nan kote ke li te ye a pou ede mwen respire si mwen ta vini genyen yon pwoblèm. Yo te fini pa retire tiyo a epi mwen te sispann bat kò mwen. Yo te voye mwen nan sal swen entansif pou mwen te kapab refè. Lè doktè yo ta va deside ke mwen te ale byen yo ta va mete mwen nan sal pou moun ki sot fè operasyon pandan yo ap tann ke yo refè epi apre yo ta va janbe mwen nan chanb lopital pou moun ki miyò. Yo te ban mwen medikaman pou soule mwen, mwen pa te byen konprann sa ki te ap pase mwen apre plizyè jou nan swen entansif la mwen te rann mwen kont ke mwen gen bagay ki pa te sa yo te dwe ye. Te gen pwoblèm, pandan ke mwen te nan sal operasyon a kè mwen pa te mache tout swit apre ke yo te koupe li a, epi pati nan kò mwen yo ki andedan vant mwen a pa te mache byen tou. Ren mwen yo te bloke. Jan pou mwen ta di sa se ke mwen te ap mouri dousman epi pèsonn pa te konnen sa pou yo te fè pou geri mwen. Mwen te swete ke mwen te kapab di Marianne adye mwen prale. Mwen te vle ke li te kouche bò kote mwen pou mwen te kapab anbrase li tout pandan ke mwen tap ale nan peyi san chapo. Mwen te vle ke dènye mo mwen yo ta di konsa : « Mwen renmen ou Marianne » Apre sa, nan lannwit la mwen te leve egare anba mòfin ak yon dekourajman nan kò mwen ak pitye pou tèt mwen. Mwen vire pou mwen peze sonèt la pou mwen rele enfimyè a epi pandan mwen ap gade pòt la, menm moman an mwen fè vizyon yon figi tou nwa san je ak bouch ki te pandye anba yon kagoul. Lè sa a mwen te ap mande tèt mwen si zanj lanmò a te vini pran nanm mwen. Apre senk jou, mwen pa te refè ase jan ke mwen te sipoze refè, kidonk doktè yo deside pou yo fè yon tès ki rele CAT SCAN pou yo ka gade tout pati ki andedan kòf lestomak mwen ak vant mwen. Se te yon jou frèt nan mwa janvye lè yo te mennen mwen al fè tès la, lè sa a mwen te ap tranble san kontwòl. Yo roule mwen nan sal tès la epi yo pran tèlman foto kò mwen ke mwen te kapab klere nan fè nwa tankou yon koukouy. Yo te voye mwen tounen nan chanb mwen pou mwen tann rezilta tès la ki te ap pare nan jou anapre a. Lè doktè a vini nan chanb mwen a li pa te poukont li, li te mennen ak li yon doktè espesyalist ki okipe maladi kansè. Li di ke yo te jwenn yon gwo timè bòkote ren mwen epi ke yo te ap bezwen retire li depi ke mwen te fè yon ale mye pou mwen te kapab sipote yon lòt operasyon. Doktè a te di mwen ke timè a te chita sou yon gwo venn epi li te ap peze venn la sa kite lakòz mwen te genyen yon maladi ki rele Deep Vein Thrombosis (DVT) Sa vle di ke venn ki enpòtan anpil andedan kò moun bouche ak san kaye. Sa te kapab lakòz ke mwen vini malad pi grav oswa ke mwen mouri. Sèl bon nouvèl ki te genyen nan pawòl maldi sa a, se ke timè a te genyen yon sak tout otou li, sa ki vle di ke mwen te kapab pran yon souf avan mwen fè operasyon a, men sa pa te vle di ke mwen te kapab tann jouk mayi mi.

Yo pa konnen pou ki rezon, men mwen te komanse refè apre yo te fè tès CAT SCAN la epi ke yo te voye mwen tounen nan chanb mwen kote mwen te rete kouche pou di jou ankò. Mwen te kontinye myò pou preske tout bagay eksepte ke mwen te genyen pwoblèm lè ke mwen te ap mache.Enfimyè a te te ede mwen leve mache nan koulwa lopital la plizyè fwa pa jou jouktan mwen te refè ase pou operasyon nan kè a te geri.

Mwen tap refè ap pran fòs lakay mwen san ke mwen pa te chaje tèt mwen pou lòt operasyon ke mwen tap pral oblije fè a. Yon zanmi mwen Diane te rete ak mwen nan kay la kòm yon enfimyè ki te domi leve. Li ede mwen pase mizè mwen. Mwen pa te kab domi byen mwen pa te manje byen tou. Okenn manje pa te gen gou nan bouch mwen. Okenn manje pa te vo lapenn ke mwen te manje li.Apre twa semen ke mwen te lakay mwen mwen tombe malad ankò epi mwen tounen lopital la. Li sanble ke ren mwen te sispan mache. Mwen pa konnen sa ki te pase, sèlman mwen te tounen lakay mwen pou mwen kontinye refè epi mwen te eseye pran ase fòs pou mwen te kapab al fè prochen operasyon a. Mwen mande si Marianne te konnen jan ke mwen te renmen li epi ki jan ke li te domaje kè mwen byen fò.

De mwa te pase apre ke mwen te fini fè operasyon kè a mwen te retounen lopital la pou yo te retire kansè a. Timè a te tèlman gwo ke se pa devan ke yo te fann mwen pou retire li. Yo te koupe mwen anpil nan operasyon sa a men mwen pa te fè okenn konplikasyon. Mwen te komanse refè preske tou swit apre operasyon a epi di jou apre mwen te tounen lakay mwen. Mwen te kontinye ap refè dousman, Diane te oblije kite mwen pou li al okipe zafè fanmi, li kidonk yon kanmarad travay mwen nan depatmen lasante a te di mwen ke mwen te kapab rete ak li ak madanm li jouktan mwen te refè ase pou mwen te kapab okipe tèt mwen poukont mwen. Mwen te pase twa semen ak kanmarad travay la. Mwen te tounen lakay mwen epi mwen te kapab vire tounen nan kay la menm ke mwen pa tap refè byen. Mwen pa te sou bò refè, mwen pa te sou sa. Mwen te ap mande mwen si sa te vo lapenn pou mwen refè. Lavi a pa te di mwen anyen.

Mwen te pase twòp tribilasyon, mwen te pran twòp lapenn. Twòp desepsyon, kounye a kò mwen te an movèzeta. Pouki sa mwen te ap pase tray sa a ? Mwen pa te jwen yon rezon pou mwen te kontinye eseye refè.

Mwen te fè yon vwayaj nan oto pou mwen te ale vizite paran mwen ki te rete 50 mil de kote ke mwen te ap viv la. Mwen pa te finn kwè ke mwen te kapab kondwi lwen konsa men mwen te deside pou mwen eseye. Mwen rive lakay paran mwen yo, mwen te bouke anpil apre ke mwen te kondwi anpil konsa. Mwen antre andedan kay la mwen bwè yon vè dlo epi mwen ale nan yon chanb ki pa te gen moun ladan li pou mwen fè yon ti domi. Lè mwen leve manman mwen te kwit manje epi li tap tann mwen. Nou te pale epi mwen te di li jan mwen te gen anpil chans de se ke mwen te vivan jodi a. Apre nou fini manje, manman mwen te ban mwen yon lèt ke yon ansyen zanmi lontan ki te fèk soti nan vwayaj te pote pou mwen. Mwen te sezi pou mwen wè ke se te Marianne ki te ekri mwen. Li ekri mwen ke li te ap eseye jwen mwen. Li ekri mwen ke li te vle eskize li pou jan ke nou te kite a. Marianne te mete tout enfòmasyon sou ki kote pou mwen te jwen li si mwen te vle pale ak li oswa rankontre li.

Mwen te fache anpil. Tout souvni lanmou nou a te disparèt tèlman mwen te an kòlè. Mwen te vle rele sou li an menm tan ke mwen te vle anbrase li fò. Mwen te realize ke mwen te ap pyafe nan kay paran mwen yo epi mwen chita pou mwen eseye kalme mwen.

Mwen li lèt la plizyè fwa pou mwen konprann vrèman sa li te vle di mwen. Mwen mete lèt la nan pòch mwen pou mwen kapab li li lè mwen tounen lakay mwen. Mwen li lèt la mwen reli li plizyè fwa menm ke mwen pa te kapab retire nan tèt mwen ke te genyen plis ke sa ki te ekri sou papye a. Menm nwit la, mwen reponn lèt li a pou mwen di li ke mwen te ap viv yon lòt kote epi ke mwen te pran yon promosyon. Mwen ekri li ke kè mwen te kontan pou jan ke lavi mwen te ap pase a. Mwen di li ke mwen te genyen yon menaj tou nèf ki te soti nan peyi Lafrans ki te gen afeksyon pou mwen. Ke menaj sa a te rete ak mwen pandan tout maladi mwen a. Mwen ekri anpil sou mwen ak menaj nèf sa a. Mwen te vele pou Marianne te konnen ke mwen pa te bezwen li ankò. Mwen menm te mete anba lèt la avan mwen siyen li sensèman. Yon fwa nan vi mwen lè ke mwen te genyen yon bagay enpòtan pou mwen te regle mwen te kite kòlè mwen pran plas santiman mwen yo. Mwen voye lèt la ale epi se tout.

De jou apre telefòn la sonnen, machin ki make nimewo moun ki ap rele a montre ke se te Marianne, mwen te kite telefòn la sonnen plizyè fwa epi mwen fòse tèt mwen reponn telefòn la. Mwen tande vwa li, tout kòlè mwen a te kaba epi mwen te pran krye. Mwen konnen ke mwen te renmen li toujou kòm si anyen pa te janm pase. Marianne eskize li pou sa ki te pase a. Li aprann mwen ke manman li te malad grav lè ke li te vle retounen vinn jwen mwen epi ke manman li te vinn mouri byen vit apre sa. Mwen te tande li ap krye tou dousman nan telefòn la lè li te ap di mwen ke li pa te janm sispan renmen mwen. Li di mwen ke li toujou kwè ke yon jou nou va tounen ansanb. Pandan ke li te ap kontinye mwen rann mwen kont ke li pa te janm abandone mwen. Marianne te ban mwen kè li. Li pa te janm reprann li.

Mwen mande li pou li padone mwen paske mwen te manke gen konfyans nan jan ke li te renmen mwen a. Nou te pale pandan lontan. Lè ke nou wè ke nou te pale ase mwen te mande li sa ke li te vle fè kounye a. Eske nou te kapab rankontre yon kote ? Li di mwen ke li te fèk fè operasyon pou kansè tou epi ke li pa tap ka vwayaje lwen. Nou te deside pou nou te rankontre nan Valdosta, Georgia. Kèk semen apre nou te rankontre. Lè sa a si yon moun ta wè nou tout le de ansanb li ta kab pran sezisman. Mwen pa te kapab soti nan machin nan poukont mwen, Marianne poukont pa li te megri tèlman ke mwen pa tap rekonèt li si mwen te wè li ap pase nan lari

a. Nou tou de te fè pitye pou moun gade. Marianne te ede mwen sòti nan oto a. Nou anbrase, nou bo, epi nou konnen ke nou ta pral rete ansanb pou tout rès lavi nou.

Nou te rankontre nan Valdosta an plizyè fwa. Mwen te ap refè pi plis chak jou. Nou te ap fè pwojè pou nou viv ansanb. Nan dènye vwayaj nou nou te ale gade nan San Mateo, Florida yon kay pou nou achte. Marianne te di mwen ke kay la te lèd, lè sa mwen te di li kijan nou te pral ranje kay la. Lè li antre andedan kay la li te renmen jan kay la te akeyan epi te ba li anvi rete ladan li. Mwen te konnen ke li ta pral vin rete ladan li nan yon ti kras tan. Nou tounen nan lotèl la epi nou ofri yon pri pou kay la. Nou te al abite kay la twa mwa apre. Malgre ke mwen pa te fini ak pwoblèm lasante mwen yo, mwen te konnen ke tout bagay ta pral antre nan plas yo. Yon ti kras tan avan ke nou vin viv nan kay la mwen te fè yon maladi ki te lakòz ke doktè yo te oblije soude ansanb zo nan kou mwen. Operasyon a te pase san pwoblèm epi mwen te santi ke mwen te kapab soti sou tab operasyon a pou mwen ale lakay mwen tou swit. Marianne te bòkote mwen pandan tout operasyon a epi pandan ke mwen te ap refè. Marianne te ap refè tou, li te ap pran yon ti repo nan lavi mouvmante li a. Li te fè yon ti gwosi epi li te rekòmanse ap souri. Mwen te kontan ke li te kapab ap refè an menm tan ak mwen.

Sipoze sa kip pase? Twa mwa apre sa mwen te fè yon lòt operasyon ankò. Yo te retire vezikil bilyè mwen !

Nan kenz mwa kat operasyon epi de kè ki repare.

Kounye a lè ke mwen ap antre nan biwo WIC la mwen ap krye tèlman mwen kontan lè ke mwen ap di Diane rès istwa a. Mwen menm ak Marianne nou kontan nan maryaj nou. Yo ban mwen yon promosyon nan pozisyon moun ki antèt pou fè travay depatman lasante a mache. Marianne fè li sitwayen Ameriken. Nou tou le de refè nèt epi nou pa gen kansè nan kò nou depi senkan.

Nou menm ak lanmou nou te kontinye ap viv.

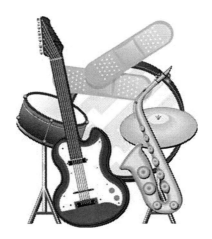

The Band-Aid

By Tracie L. Dickerson

Over my summer vacation I discovered just how important a band-aid could be. Working for the Health Department and attending all of the extra trainings has made me more prepared for minor emergencies. Before embarking on a 3,000 mile journey through Nevada, California, Arizona and Utah I decided that I should get some water and other provisions, considering the sweltering 117 degrees it was outside. I went to the front desk the evening before to get two important things, 1. the directions to the local mega-mart and 2. the directions to Death Valley National Park.As the Concierge was looking for my directions a slightly panicked and very frantic person ran up to the counter. She exclaimed, "Someone has been hurt. It's not too bad but he may need stitches. I am a nurse and I need a butterfly band-aid." The concierge looks to me and asks again where I was planning to travel to. I was perplexed. A paying guest took precedence over a minor emergency! I looked at this nicely dressed woman and looked back at the front desk help. Understanding the needs of a bleeding person that may need stitches came well before my directions to Death Valley, I told the front desk person to find the first aid kit.

I learned long ago that the donut glazed over eyes with the blank faced stare is never something you want to see from a person who is supposed to help you. To my utter shock and surprise the clerk walked away and went to the back for what seemed like an eternity.

I spoke with the frazzled woman to help her calm down a bit. I discovered that her boyfriend was the bass player in a band that was playing at the hotel bar. Some equipment fell and he had a two inch gash on his forehead. Cancelling the concert was not an option, but forehead wounds bleed like crazy and she needed to do something quickly.

We waited a few more moments for the clerk to return. "I am sorry miss, but we don't have a first aid kit". Realizing that the moment needed some decisive action, I switched into lawyer mode. "You mean the front desk does not have a first-aid kit?" He responded with a "Yes." Does housekeeping have a first aid kit? "No", do the employees have a first aid kit? No. If you fell and hurt yourself who would you call? Security.

Aha! So security was the answer to getting the person help. So security might have a band-aid? Yes. Some of the guards have been EMT trained.

"Great," I said, you call security and have them report to the café with the band-aids.

In an abundance of caution, I always carry a small first aid kit with me when I travel. I have used it only once, but I feel better knowing it is there. I looked at the woman and said, "I have a first-aid kit in my room. It is small, but at least it is something. I will meet you at the café." Dashing up to my room, I went over to my carry on and after a few seconds of searching I found my trusty kit. I went back downstairs and on the way saw the security guard that had been dispatched with his one band-aid.

The security guard saw me and told me to go back to my room. I headed back toward the elevator, but then my Health Department trainings kicked in. I knew what I needed to do. At the very least I needed to find the woman and let her know that I had come back. I needed to make sure that I was no longer a necessary part of the equation!

After three times through the concepts of Incident Command training and the importance of making sure I was not needed, Security let me into the Club/Café. Within seconds I found the woman. She was still in distress! The Security Guard was unable to help her boyfriend, who was now on stage playing. The large (still bleeding) gash on his head was mostly covered by a folded napkin sandwiched in by a large hat.

When I handed over my first-aid kit complete with alcohol swabs and butterfly band-aids, I thought this woman was going to cry. She gave me a huge hug, bought me a drink and invited me to stay as a guest of the band for the rest of the night. It makes me laugh to think that I was a band aid for the evening!

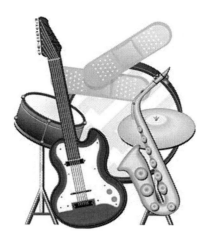

La Curita

Por Tracie L. Dickerson

En mis vacaciones de verano descubrí lo importante que una curita podía ser. Trabajar para el departamento de salud y atender a los entrenamientos extras me han preparado más para emergencias menores. Antes de embarcarme a un viaje de 3,000 millas a través de Nevada, California, Arizona y Utah, decidí que yo debía llevar algo de agua y otras provisiones, considerando los ardientes 117 grados de temperatura que hacía afuera. Fui a la recepción la noche anterior a fin de obtener dos cosas importantes, 1. Direcciones de cómo llegar a la tienda por departamento de la localidad y 2. Direcciones de cómo llegar a Death Valley National Park.

Mientras el conserje estaba buscando las direcciones una persona con cierto pánico y muy ansiosa se acercó a la recepción. Ella exclamó, "Alguien se ha lesionado. No es tan grave pero puede necesitar puntos. Yo soy una enfermera y necesito una curita en forma de mariposa." El empleado me mira a mí y pregunta otra vez a dónde es que yo planeo viajar.

Yo estaba perpleja. ¡Una visitante que estaba pagando tomaba precedente sobre una emergencia menor! Yo miré a esa mujer que muy decentemente vestía y miré de nuevo al escritorio de atención al cliente. Entendiendo que las necesidades de una persona que sangraba y podía necesitar puntos eran más importantes que las direcciones de cómo llegar a Death Valley, yo le dije al empleado de servicio al cliente que encontrara el equipo de primeros auxilios.

Yo aprendí hace mucho tiempo atrás que la mirada sostenida congelada y sorprendida con cara apática es algo que tú nunca quieres ver de una persona que se supone debe ayudarte. Para mi mayor asombro y sorpresa el empleado se retiró hacia atrás lo cual pareció una eternidad.

Yo hablé con la descompuesta mujer a fin de ayudarla a calmarse. Descubrí que su novio era el que tocaba el bajo de la banda que estaba tocando en el bar del hotel. Algún equipo se cayó y tuvo una abertura de dos pulgadas en su frente. Cancelar el concierto no era una opción, pero las aberturas de frente sangran bastante y ella necesitaba hacer algo rápido.

Esperamos unos momentos más a fin de que el empleado regresara. "Lo siento señorita, pero nosotros no tenemos un equipo de primeros auxilios." Dándome cuenta que se necesitaba una acción decisiva, me conecté con mi estilo de abogado, "¿Usted quiere decir que el escritorio de atención al cliente no tiene un equipo de primeros auxilios?" Él respondió con un "Sí". "¿Tiene el Departamento de Mantenimiento un equipo de primeros auxilios?" "No". "¿Si tú te caes y te lastimas a quién llamarías?" "A Seguridad."

¡Aha! Seguridad era la respuesta para proporcionar ayuda a la persona. "¿Entonces, Seguridad debe tener una curita?"

"Sí. Algunos de los guardias están entrenados en EMT."

"Maravilloso. Tú llamas a Seguridad y haces que ellos se reporten al Café con una curita".

Con abundancia de precaución, yo siempre llevo conmigo un pequeño equipo de primeros auxilios cuando viajo. Lo he usado solo una vez, pero me siento mejor sabiendo que esta allí. Yo miré a la mujer y le dije, "Yo tengo un maletín de primeros auxilios en mi cuarto. Es pequeño, pero al menos es algo. Me encontraré contigo en el Café." Subí corriendo a mi cuarto, revisé una maleta de rodar y después de buscar por unos segundos encontré mi valioso maletín de primeros auxilios. Regresé abajo y en la vía vi al guardia de seguridad que había sido despachado con una curita.

El guardia de seguridad me vio y me dijo que me regresara a mi cuarto. Me regresé al elevador, pero luego mis entrenamientos del Departamento de Salud se activaron. Sabía lo que debía hacer.

Por lo menos, tenía que encontrar a la mujer y decirle que yo había regresado. ¡Tenía que estar segura de que ya yo no era una parte indispensable de la ecuación!

Después de pasar tres veces por los conceptos del Entrenamiento de Comando de Incidente y la importancia de estar segura que no era necesitada, Seguridad me dejó entrar al Club/Café. En unos segundos encontré a la mujer. ¡Ella estaba todavía angustiada! El Guardia de Seguridad no había podido ayudar a su novio, quien estaba ahora sobre la tarima tocando. La gran (todavía sangrante) herida estaba mayormente cubierta por una servilleta doblada, la cual parecía formar el relleno de un sándwich, sostenida por un gran sombrero.

Cuando le entregué mi equipo de primeros auxilios completo con toallitas con alcohol y curitas en forma de mariposa, yo pensé que esa mujer iba a llorar. Me dio un gran abrazo, me trajo algo de tomar y me invitó a quedarme como invitada de la banda por el resto de la noche. ¡Me da risa pensar que yo fui una band-aid por esa noche!

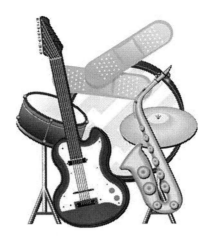

Pansman A

Se Tracie L. Dickerson ki ekri istwa sa a.

Pandan vakans mwen pran nan mwa gran vakans yo, mwen te dekouvri kijan yon ti pansman te enpòtan. Kòm mwen travay ak depatman lasante a epi mwen te asiste tout seminè fòòmasyon yo mwen pi byen pare pou ti ka ijans. Avan ke mwen anbake nan yon vwayaj nan oto ki sou 3000mil pase nan Nevada, California, Arizonna ak Utah. Mwen te deside pou mwen al achete dlo ak lòt provizyon tèlman te fè cho. Yon tanperati de 117 degre deyò a. Mwen ale nan biwo lotèl la kote yo resevwa moun, kote mwen te mande de enfòmasyon. 1) Ki jan pou mwen ale nan gwo sipèmakèt nan zòn nan 2). Ki jan pou mwen ale nan Pak nasyonal nan Death Valley.

Pandan moun ki travay nan biwo resepsyon an tap chache enfòmasyon pou mwen, yon fi ajite ak laperèz nan kò li kouri vini devan kontwa lotèl la. Li rapote ke gen yon moun ki blese, pa twò grav. Men li bezwen ke yo koude blesi a. Mwen se yon enfimyè mwen bezwen pansman ki fèt tankou papiyon yo pou fèmen blesi a pou moun nan. Moun ki te sou biwo a gade m epi li mande-m ankò ki kote mwen vle al flannen a.

Sa te twouble mwen pou mwen wè yon envite lotèl pi enpòtan que yon ka ijans. Mwen gade madam nan ki te byen abiye epi mwen vire gade anplwaye a. Kòm mwen te konprann ke li te pi enpòtan pou yo te okipe moun ki te blese a, ke pou yo te di mwen ki jan pou mwen te fè pou mwen te ale nan pak Death Valley a. Mwen di anplwaye a pou li okipe chèche bwat ki geyen materyèl pansman pou ka ijans yo.

Depi lontan mwen konnen ke ou pa janm renmen wè moun ki dwe ede fè je li tankou je pwason fri, epi mete figi li lwen tankou moun ki nan lalin. Mwen sezi jouk mwen pa konnen lè anplwaye a ale nan pyès deyè kontwa a epi li rete yon pakèt tan, yon etènite.

Mwen pale ak fi a ki te ajite a pou li kalme li yon ti kras. Mwen dekouvri ke menaj li te jwe bas nan djaz ki te jwe mizik nan ba lotèl la. Te genyen yon ekipman ki te tombe sou tèt li epi fwon li te koupe ak yon blesi de pous. Yo pa te kapab ranvwaye konsè a. Men blesi nan fwon senyen anpil epi li te bezwen fè san ki te ap koule a sispan koule byen vit.

Nou tann yon bon moman pou anplwaye biwo lotèl la tounen. Lè li tounen li di : » Mwen regrèt anpil madam men nou pa gen bwat ki geyen materyèl pansman pou ka ijans" Lè mwen te wè ke lè sa yon moun te dwe pran yon desizyon pou fè bagay mache, mwen kòmanse pale kòm si mwen se te yon avoka epi mwen di li:" Ou vle di mwen ke biwo lotèl la pa genyen bwat ki geyen materyèl pansman pou ka ijans"? Li reponn mwen "wi " Mwen mande li: » Eske moun ki reskonsab pou kenbe lotèl la pwòp pa gen yon bwat ki geyen materyèl pansman pou ka ijans"? "Non" Si ou ta va tombe epi ou ta va blese ki moun ke ou ap rele? "Sekirite"

Aha! Kidonk se sekirite ki solisyon pou nou jwen yon jan pou ede moun blese a. Kidonk se sekirite ki kapab ba nou pansman a.

"Wi genyen kèk nan sekirite gad yo ki te ale nan antrenman pou sekouris"

"Bèl bagay, " Mwen di li " Rele sekirite epi di gad la pou li vini nan kafeterya lotèl ak pansman a.

Kòm mwen se yon moun ki renmen pran anpil prekosyon, depi ke mwen ap vwayaje mwen toujou mache ak yon twous ki geyen materyèl pou ka ijans. Mwen te sèvi ak bwat twoua sa a yon sèl fwa sèlman, men mwen toujou santi mwen pi an sekirite lè ke mwen gen twous ijans la ak mwen. Mwen gade madanm nan epi mwen di li:"Mwen gen yon twoua ki geyen materyèl pou ka ijans nan chanb mwen. Li piti men omwens na gen yon bagay pou ede ak blesi a. Map vin jwen ou nan kafeterya lotèl la. " wen plonje al nan chanb mwen, mwen pran ti malèt piti moun pote adedan avyon yo epi apre ke mwen chèche pandan kèk segond mwen jwen twous la ki konnen ban mwen konfyans la. Mwen desann anba nan lotèl la epi pandan mwen ap mache a mwen wè sekirite a ke yo te voye ak yon grenn pansman.

Sekirite gad la wè mwen epi li di mwen pou mwen tounen al nan chanb mwen. Mwen vire pou mwen ale nan asansè lotèl la, men antrenman yo ban mwen nan depatman lasante a fè mwen reflechi. Mwen te konnen sa mwen te dwe fè. Omwens fòk mwen te jwenn ak madam la epi fè li konnen ke mwen te retounen vinn jwenn li jan mwen te di li a. Mwen te vle asire mwen tou ke yo pa te bezwen mwen ankò nan sa ki te ap pase a. Apre ke mwen te ale twa fwa nan seminè sou ki jan pou moun aji lè ke genyen yon pwoblèm epi ke mwen te aprann ki jan li enpòtan pou mwen toujou asire mwen ke yo pa te bezwen mwen tout bon vre mwen mache al nan kafeterya a. Sekirite gad la te kite mwen antre nan kafetrya a. Apre yon segond mwen te jwen madanm la. Li pa te sispan bat kò li akòz de pwoblèm la. Sekirite gad la pa te kapab ede menaj li a ki te ap jwe mizik sou sèn la. Yo te kouvri gwo blesi nan fwon li a ak yon napron an papye ke yon chapo te kenbe.

Lè mwen lonje bay madanm la bwat ki geyen materyèl pou ka ijans la ki te genyen aplikatè mouye ak alkòl ansanb ak pansman an fòm papiyon, mwen te kwè ke madanm la ta pral kòmanse krye. Li anbrase mwen byen fò,li achte yon bwason pou mwen bwè epi li envite mwen pou mwen rete pandan tout lannwit la kòm envite djaz la. Li fè mwen ri lè mwen sonje ke mwen se te yon pansman ki te anpeche pwogram mizik lannwit la gate! ☀

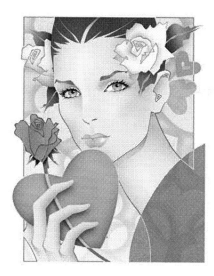

The Greatest Gift

By Mort Laitner

My office phone rang six times before I picked up the receiver. I heard my mother's familiar voice. Something was wrong. Her words trembled, "Son, I got my test results. My doctor said I have pancreatic cancer!" My heart fell to the floor. Fear paralyzed my body. Tears formed in my eyes then rolled down my face. I tasted salt as these tears ran onto my lips.

"Mom, you'll be okay. You'll beat it. You are a survivor." What else could I say? The words left my mouth in a quiver. "I'll see you tonight. We'll work on a plan. I'll start researching the disease. I love you, good bye."

As I hung up the phone, I realized I knew absolutely nothing about pancreatic cancer. Immediately, I started an internet search. I read twenty sites in two hours. What I learned was not encouraging. In article after article, one number kept hitting me – six. Each site said that a person diagnosed with pancreatic cancer had only 6 months left to live. I studied the experimental treatments; all of them were a million to one.

My mother and I visited Baptist Hospital for her weekly chemotherapy. Mom was willing to be a human guinea pig in exchange for additional days on earth. I became her chauffeur, her entertainer and her cheerer-upper. While the injected chemo flowed into her veins, I read her stories. We reminisced about the good old days with our family and friends.

Mom lived on hope. She believed as a survivor that she could fight any disease and win. After three months of chemo, Mom scheduled her oncologist appointment. We would learn if the therapy was working. We took our usual drive to Baptist, silently praying for the success of the experimental therapy. As I looked at my mother sitting in the doctor's waiting room, she looked nervous but extremely hopeful. The young oncologist called us into his office and stood as he matter-of-factly looked at my mother and said, "Sorry, the experimental treatment failed." He then followed, "There is nothing else we can do to extend your life." I felt a hard fist punch into my solar plexus. The air was knocked out of my body. I looked at my mom's face. She held back her tears but she aged ten years in front of my eyes. Mom's hope had vanished. As I left the doctor's office and walked though the hospital to get to the garage, I cried uncontrollably. I did not care if anyone noticed. I pulled myself together by the time I drove to the front of the hospital to pick up Mom. We silently drove back to her home, each of us wondering why our prayers went unanswered.

I watched my mother deteriorate.

I had studied, "On Death and Dying" during the early days of the AIDS crisis. I decided to reread Kübler-Ross's classic. I watched as Mom journeyed through each of the five stages of loss – denial, anger, bargaining, depression, and, finally, acceptance.

As the cancer shriveled up my mother, my sister and I were advised to bring in a hospice worker. This angel of mercy gave us the comfort and assurance that we would survive this ordeal. My sister and I decided to rotate nights taking care of Mom. The night before my mother passed away, she suffered terribly. The pain caused angry words to be spewed at my sister. The next morning, I heard about the horrible night and was thankful that I was spared listening to my mother's agony. The doctor ordered an increase in morphine drops to numb the pain and to put Mom on a no-food-or-liquid regime. The hospice worker opined, "I think this will be your mother's last day with us." I calculated the dates, exactly six months from that fateful telephone call. That night I held Mom's hands in mine. Trembling, I said, "I'm going to miss you so much. Say hi to Dad for me. I love you." And my mom uttered her last three words, "I love you." Within an hour Mom passed away. My sister and I cried like abandoned orphans.

Eight years have passed since the death watch. I think of Mom on a daily basis, realizing that her parting words were the greatest gift she ever gave me.

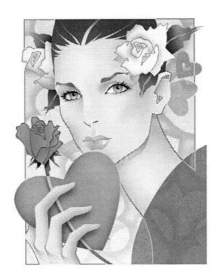

El Mejor Regalo

Por Mort Laitner

El teléfono de mi oficina sonó tres veces antes de que yo lo respondiera. Oí la voz familiar de mi madre. Algo andaba mal. Su voz tembló, "!Hijo, me dieron los resultados de los exámenes. Mi doctor dice que yo tengo cáncer del páncreas!" Mi corazón se cayó al suelo. Lágrimas llenaron mis ojos y luego rodaron sobre mi cara. Yo saboreé la sal mientras estas lágrimas corrían sobre mis labios.

"Mamá, tú estarás bien. Lo combatirás. Tú eres una sobreviviente." ¿Qué más podía yo decir? Mis palabras salieron de mi boca temblando. "Te veré esta noche. Trazaremos un plan. Yo empezaré a investigar sobre la enfermedad. Te quiero, chao."

Al cerrar el teléfono, me di cuenta que no sabía absolutamente nada sobre el cáncer de páncreas. Inmediatamente, comencé a investigar en el Internet. Leí veinte páginas web en dos horas. Lo que aprendí no era esperanzador. Artículo tras artículo un número se mantenía pegándome – seis. Cada página web decía que una persona a quien se le diagnosticara cáncer pancreático tenía solo seis meses de vida. Yo estudié los tratamientos experimentales; todos ellos era uno en un millón.

Mi Mamá y yo visitamos el Baptist Hospital para su quimioterapia semanal. Mi Mamá estaba dispuesta a ser conejillo de india a cambio de algunos días adicionales sobre la tierra. Me volví su chofer, entretenedor y su alzador del espíritu. Mientras la inyectada quimioterapia corría sobre sus venas, yo leía sus historias. Recordamos los maravillosos viejos días con familia y amigos.

Mamá vivía en esperanza. Ella creyó como superviviente que podía combatir cualquier enfermedad y ganar. Después de tres meses de quimioterapia, Mamá programó su cita con el oncólogo. Sabríamos si la terapia estaba funcionando. Hicimos nuestro usual viaje al Baptist, silenciosamente rezando por el éxito de la terapia experimental. Mientras miraba a mi mamá en la sala de espera del doctor, ella se veía nerviosa pero con mucha esperanza. El joven oncólogo nos llamó a su oficina y se paró mirando a mi mamá y dijo, "Lo siento, el tratamiento experimental falló." Luego dijo, "No hay más nada que podamos hacer para extenderle la vida." Sentí un duro golpe de puño en mi plexo solar. El aire fue sacado de mi cuerpo. Yo miré la cara de mi mamá. Ella aguantó sus lágrimas pero envejeció diez años enfrente de mis ojos. Las esperanzas de mi Mamá se desvanecieron. Mientras salía de la oficina del doctor y caminaba a través del hospital para llegar al garaje, lloré incontrolablemente. No me importó si alguien lo notaba. Yo me contuve un poco al momento en el que manejé al frente del hospital a buscar a mi Mamá. Regresamos silenciosamente a su casa, preguntándonos por qué nuestras oraciones no fueron contestadas.

Vi como mi mamá se deterioraba.

Yo he estudiado, "Sobre la Muerte y Muriendo" durante los primeros días de la crisis del SIDA. Yo decidí releer el clásico de Kübler-Ross. Yo pude ver como mi Mamá pasaba a través de los cinco estados de pérdida – negación, rabia, entendimiento, depresión, y, finalmente, aceptación.

Mientras el cáncer consumía el cuerpo de mi madre, mi hermana y yo fuimos aconsejados a traer un trabajador médico de enfermedades terminales. Este ángel de misericordia nos dio la consolación y la seguridad de que nosotros sobreviviríamos esta odisea. Mi hermana y yo decidimos turnarnos las noches a fin cuidar a Mamá. La noche anterior a su muerte, ella sufrió terriblemente. El dolor causó que ella le lanzara palabras enfadadas a mi hermana. A la mañana siguiente, oí sobre la terrible noche y di gracias que yo fui liberado de oír la agonía de mi madre. El doctor ordenó un incremento en las gotas de morfina para eliminar el dolor y puso a Mamá en un régimen de no comer ni beber. El trabajador médico opinó, "Creo que este será el último día de vuestra Mamá con nosotros." Calculé las fechas, exactamente seis meses de esa desafortunada llamada telefónica. Esa noche yo agarré las manos de Mamá con las mías. Temblando, le dije, "Te voy a extrañar tanto. Dile hola a papá de mi parte. Te quiero." Y mi mamá pronunció sus tres últimas palabras, "Yo te quiero." Durante la hora siguiente Mamá murió. Mi hermana y yo lloramos como huérfanos abandonados.

Ocho años han pasado desde que presencié la muerte. Pienso en Mamá diariamente, dándome cuenta que sus palabras de partida fueron el mejor regalo que ella alguna vez me hizo.

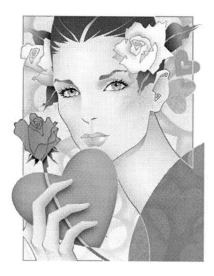

Pi gwo kado a

Se Mort Laitner ki ekri istwa sa a.
Mwen sonje ou manman

Telefòn nan biwo mwen sonnen sis fwa avan ke mwen pran li. Mwen rekonèt vwa manman mwen. Te genyen yon bagay ki tap pase. Li tranble lè li ap di mo sa yo, «Pitit gason mwen, yo ban mwen rezilta tès mwen yo. Doktè a di mwen ke mwen genyen kansè nan pankrea mwen «Se te tankou kè mwen te tonbe a tè. La-perèz te paralize kò mwen. Dlo te plen je mwen, epi li tap koule sou figi mwen. Mwen goute sèl ki te nan krye a lè dlo nan je mwen te rive nan bouch mwen.

«Manman ou ap byen. Ou ap genyen batay la. Ou se yon moun ki konnen lite ou ap siviv li.» Ki lòt bagay ke mwen te kapab di ? Mo yo soti nan bouch mwen ki tap tramble «Na wè aswè a. Na va travay sou yon plan. Mwen ap pral komanse fè rechèch sou maladi a. Mwen renmen ou, m'ale»

Pandan ke mwen ap fèmen telefòn la, mwen rann mwen kont ke mwen pa te konnen anyen di tou sou kansè nan pankrea. Menm moman, mwen ale nan entènèt pou mwen fè rechèch. Mwen li ven sit entènèt nan de zè de tan. Sa mwen te aprannn la pa te ankourajan di tou. Mwen pase papye rechèch ekri apre paye rechèch ekri sou maladi a, a chak fwa te genyen yon nimewo ki kontinye ap frape mwen –sis. Chak sit entènèt ke mwen te li te di ke yon moun ke doktè dyagnostike ak kansè nan pankrea rete sèlman sis mwa pou li viv. Mwen etidye trètman kote yo ap fè eksperyans pou wè nan yo sa ki mache, nan tout tretman yo, chans yo te yon milyon chans pou moun nan mouri pou yon sèl chans pou moun nan viv.

Manman mwen avèk mwen nou ale nan lopital Baptist Hospital pou li te ale pran tretman chimik pou kansè ke li te ap prann chak semen la. Pou ke li te kapab viv kèk jou ankò sou latè, manman mwen te aksepte pou yo fè eksperyans sou li tankou yo fè sou ti bèt kochon dend nan laboratwa. Mwen te tounen chofè li, moun ki ap distrè li, moun ki ap remonte moral li. Pandan yo tap mete pwodwi chimik nan venn li, mwen te li istwa pou li. Ansanb nou te sonje bon vye tan lontan ke nou te pase ak zanmi ak fanmi.

Manman mwen te ap viv ak espwa. Li te kwè ke kòm yon moun ki konnen lite pou la vi li eki te toujou kon genyen batay yo, li tap kapab goumen ak nenpòt maladi epi pote la viktwa. Apre twa mwa ap prann tretman ak pwodwi chimik, manman mwen te fè randevou ak doktè espesyalist kansè yo rele onkologist. Nou tap pral konnen si tretman a tap mache. Kòm dabitid nou chita nan oto mwen tap konduyi a pou nou ale lopital Baptist la, lè sa a nou tap lapryè an silans pou ke tretman kote yo ap fè eksperyans la ta va mache. Lè mwen tap gade manman mwen ki te chita nan sal atant doktè a, li te sanble ke malgre ke kè li tap sote li te gen anpil lespwa. Jenn doktè espesyalist kansè a rele nou nan biwo li, li kanpe epi san fason kareman li gade manman mwen epi li di» Mwen regrèt pou mwen di ou ke tretman kote yo ap fè eksperyans la pa mache «epi tou li kontinye di nou» Pa gen anyen ankò nou kapab fè pou ke ou kontinye viv pi lontan» Mwen santi se te kòm si yon moun te ban mwen yon kout pwen anba biskèt mwen .Souf mwen te koupe, tout lè te soti nan kò mwen. Mwen gade figi manman mwen. Li kenbe krye li, dlo pa te sòt nan zye li, men li te vin vye granmoun menm moman a, se te kòm si dizan te ajoute sou laj li nan yon sèl moman pandan ke mwen tap gade li a. Tout lespwa manman 'm te geyen a te pèdi. Lè mwen tap kite klinik doktè a, epi ke mwen tap travèse lopital la pou mwen ale nan garaj la, mwen krye san kontwòl. Sa pa te mele mwen ke moun te wè mwen ap krye. Mwen vin ranmase karaktè mwen lè ke mwen konduyi machin la devan lopital la pou mwen te pran manman mwen. Pandan mwen tap konduyi machin la pou mennenn lakay li nou pa te di yon mo, nou chak tap made tèt nou poukisa lapryè nou pa te ekzose.

Mwen swiv jan ke eta manman mwen te ap deteryore.

Mwen te etidye sou lanmò ak moun ki ap mouri «On Death and Dying» pandan epòk lè ke katastwòf maladi Sida a te fèk kòmanse. Mwen te deside pou mwen li yon lòt fwa ankò enfomasyon moun ki rele Kübler-Ross te ekri sou moun ki ap mouri. Mwen te wè lè ke manman mwen tap travese chak nan senk etap ke moun pase lè ke yo ap pèdi lavi yo : Derefize aksepte sa ki ap pase yo a, antre an kolè, esye machande ak lanmò a, vini deprime, epi finalman aksepte sityasyon a.

Kòm manman mwen tap depafini anba kansè a, yo te bay mwen menm ak sè-m la konsèy pou nou fè yon travyè ki kon okipe moun ki ap mouri vini rete ak li. Travayè sa a se te yon zanj de mizerikòd ki te ban nou kouraj epi asire nou ke nou tap soti vivan nan move kadè nou tap pase a. Sè-m nan ak mwen nou te deside nou tap fè roulman lannwit pou okipe manman nou. Lanwit avan manman mwen trepase a, li te soufri anpil. Doulè a te lakòz ke li te deblatere pawòl moun ki ankolè bay sè-m la. Le landemen maten , mwen te tande kijan manman men te pase yon nwit terib e mwen te remesye bon dye de se ke mwen pa te oblije asiste agoni manman mwen. Doktè a bay lòd pou ogmante gout mòfin yo pou kalme doulè manman mwen yo, epi li bay lòd pou yo pa ba li ni bwè ni manje. Travyè ki konnen okipe moun ki ap mouri a di nou » Mwen kwè ke jodi a se ap dènye jou manman nou avèk nou.»Mwen kalkile dat la, se te ekzakteman si mwa depi ke mwen te resevwa kout telefòn fatal la. Nwit sa a mwen te kenbe men manman mwen nan pa mwen. Mwen tap tranble, mwen di li « Mwen ap pral manke ou anpil. Di papa mwen bonjou pou mwen. Mwen renmen ou » Epi manman mwen te soufle twa dènye mo sa yo » Mwen renmen ou.» Inè de tan apre manman mwen te mouri. Sè-m mwen a ak mwen nou krye tankou ti moun òfelen.

Sa fè ywit an ki pase depi ke mwen te asiste lanmò manman mwen Mwen sonje manman mwen chak jou, epi mwen rann mwen kont ke mo li te di mwen yo avan ke li te ale a se te pi gwo kado ke li te janm ban mwen. ✺

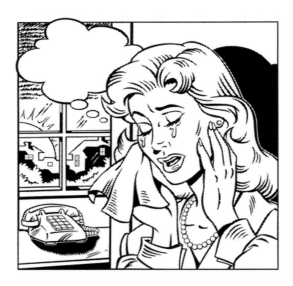

Many Healthy Stories readers have asked what response we received from the "Greatest Gift" story, here it is.

A Rivulet of Tears

By our Readers

The e-mails flowed in like a gentle stream rolling down a hill.
The story had hit a nerve, the optic nerve to be exact.
I remembered crying as I wrote it. Was it too personal to divulge?
Now others were sharing their perceptions as well as their grief.

"The story is a moving narrative of a painful chapter in life. As I read it, I remembered my mom's last days, our last word together. We each said, 'I love you'. "
Tears of love

The trickling continued, "Not a day goes by when I do not think about my mother…My old habit of calling her to say I'm OK…A moment I want to share with Mom and then remember I can't. However, I do feel her presence. She stays with me for as long as I need her. I never feel alone."
Tears of togetherness

A note from my sister, "Thanks for the morning cry. Every day I think of Mom."
Tears *of remembrance*

The next e-mail said it in just three words, "I cried too."
Tears of understanding

As I walked down the hall, a coworker approached me and said, "I loved the story and to my astonishment, I uncontrollably wept in my cubicle."
Tears *of release*

"The story brought me to tears, and it has reminded me how deep the love of a son is. That's beautiful."
Tears *of family*

"I do not know what to say. My mom passed away a year ago. I can not describe my agony. I'm not ashamed to say, 'I cried and even screamed.' I thank God for the time we had together."

Tears *of thanks*

"I'm a cancer survivor. The story meant so much to me"
Tears *of survival*

"My mother recently died and I am still recovering."
Tears *of recovery*

"I felt your sadness …and dread the day I will have to miss my mom."
Tears *of dread*

The final e-mail was heartfelt. "A son never forgets…"
Tears

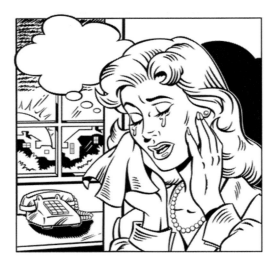

Muchos lectores de Healthy Stories nos han preguntado que respuestas hemos recibido de la historia "El Mejor Regalo," aquí están.

Un Torrente De Lágrimas

Por Nuestros Lectores

Los correos electrónicos fluyeron como un suave riachuelo cayendo por una colina. La historia le ha dado a un nervio, el nervio óptico para ser exactos.

Recuerdo llorar mientras la escribía. ¿Era muy personal para divulgarla? Ahora otros estaban compartiendo sus percepciones y penas.

La historia es una narrativa emotiva de un capítulo doloroso en la vida. Mientras la leía, me recordé de los últimos días de mi mamá, nuestras últimas palabras juntos. Cada uno dijo, "Te quiero."
Lágrimas *de amor*

La caída continuó, "No pasa un día en el cual yo no piense en mi madre...Mi viejo hábito de llamarla para decirle estoy bien...un

momento que quisiera compartir con mi Mamá y luego recuerdo que no puedo. Sin embargo, yo siento su presencia. Ella está conmigo siempre que la necesito. Nunca me siento sola."
Lágrimas de unidad

Una nota de mi hermana, "Gracias por la llorada de la mañana. Todo los días pienso en Mamá."
Lágrimas de remembranza

El siguiente e-mail lo dijo tan solo en tres palabras, "Yo lloré también."
Lágrimas de entendimiento

Mientras caminaba por el pasillo, un compañero de trabajo se acercó a mí y dijo, "Me encantó la historia y para mi asombro, lloré incontrolablemente en mi cubículo."
Lágrimas de desahogo

"La historia me llenó de lágrimas, y me ha recordado lo profundo que es el amor de un hijo. Es bellísimo."
Lágrimas de familia

"No sé que decir. Mi mamá murió hace un año. No puedo describir mi agonía. No tengo pena de decir, 'lloré e inclusive grité.' Le dio gracias a Dios por el tiempo que estuvimos juntas."
Lágrimas de agradecimiento

"Yo sobreviví el cáncer. La historia significó mucho para mí."
Lágrimas de supervivencia

"Mi madre murió hace poco y todavía me estoy recobrando."
Lágrimas de recuperación

"Sentí tu tristeza...y tengo miedo del día en el cual tenga que extrañar a mi mamá."
Lágrimas de miedo

El último correo electrónico era sincero. "Un hijo nunca olvida."
Lágrimas

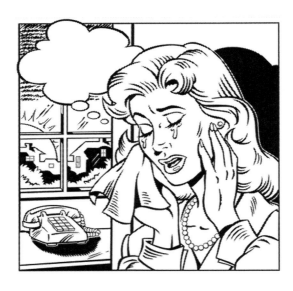

Anpil moun ki te li liv Istwa Sou Lasante te mande nou kisa moun ki te li yonn nan istwa yo ki rele " Pi Gwo Kado" te fè. Men sa yo te ekri epi di:

Krye Tankou Larivyè

Se moun ki li istwa yo ki ekri sa a.

Tout lèt moun te ekri nan konpitè yo sa yo rele e-mail tap vini tankou yon rivyè kap koule sòt sou tèt yon mòn. Istwa a te touché yon nè, nè ki nan je moun ki fè yo krye pou nou pale pi klè. Mwen sonje jan ke mwen te krye lè ke mwen te ap ekri istwa sa a. Eske istwa a te gen twòp biznis prive mwen ladan li pou ke mwen te al bay tout moun li li?

Apre ke lòt moun te finn li istwa a yo tap di nou kouman yo te santi yo lè yo tap li istwa a epi tou lapenn ke yo te genyen.

Istwa a rakonte yon epizòd nan lavi ki plen ak lapenn li ekri nan yon jan ki boulvèse moun ki li li .Pandan mwen tap li li mwen sonje dènye jou nan lavi manman mwen, dènye pawòl nou te di yon lòt, Nou chak te di:" Mwen renmen ou".

Krye akòz lanmou.

Repons yo kontinye ap vide sou nou" Pa gen yon jou ki pase san ke mwen pa sonje manman mwen. Vye abitid mwen genyen pou mwen rele li pou mwen di li ke mwen bye. Nan yon moman mwen vle rele manman mwen pou mwen fè yon ti pale ak li epi mwen vin sonje ke mwen pa kapab paske li pa la ankò. Malgre sa mwen santi ke li la ak mwen. Li rete ak mwen tout otan ke mwen bezwen li. Mwen pa janm santi mwen pou kont mwen.

Krye paske nou te ansanb.

Sè mwen a ekri mwen yon ti biye ladan li li ekri" Mèsi deske ou fè mwen krye an maten a. Chak jou ki pase mwen sonje manman nou tou.

Krye paske yo te sonje manman pa yo tou.

Lòt lèt nan konpitè a te di sa yo te santi nan twa mo sèlman (an angle) " Mwen te krye tou."

Krye paske moun nan te konprann filing mwen

Pandan mwen tap mache nan koulwa biwo a nan travay la, yon moun ki ap travay menm kote ak mwen te vini kote mwen epi li te di mwen . Mwen renmen istwa ou a epi mwen sezi lè li te di mwen:" Mwen te krye san ke mwen pa te kapab kontwole mwen, kote mwen te chita nan ti bout kwen biwo mwen a.

Krye paske moun nan te jwen soulajman

"Istwa a te fè mwen krye epi li fè mwen sonje kouman lanmou yon pitit gason pou manman li kapab anpil nan tou fon kè li. Se yon bèl bagay.

Krye paske moun nan sonje fanmi li

Mwen pa konnen sa pou mwen di. Manman mwen mouri lane pase. Mwen pa kab esplike ou nan ki agoni mwen te ye. Mwen pa wont pou mwen di ke mwen krye mwen menm rele. Mwen remèsye Bondye pou tan mwen te pase ak manman mwen.

Krye pou remèsye mwen

Mwen se yon moun ki chape anba lanmò ak maladi kansè. Istwa sa a enpòtan pou mwen.
Krye moun ki te chape anba lapenn ak pwoblèm

Manman mwen fèk mouri mwen poko refè nèt depi lanmo a.
Krye pou moun ki ap refè.

Mwen santi lapenn ou, epi mwen ap tranble pou jou mwen ta vin pèdi manmanm mwen ta vin rive sou mwen, lè sa a mwen va manke genyen manman mwen ak mwen.
Krye paske moun nan te gen lapenn.

Dènye lèt nan konpitè a tap fann kè ou" Yon pitit gason pa janm bliye."

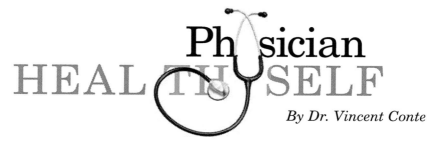

Ph sician
HEAL TH SELF

By Dr. Vincent Conte

It started as a slight nagging ache in my lower back that just wouldn't go away. Advil made it better, but still the ache would return. It worsened over the next two months until finally I stopped a neurologist colleague of mine in the hospital hallway and told him about it. He wrote me a prescription for a CAT scan and instructed me to have the results sent to his office.

The day came for my scan. It was a beautiful, sunny Wednesday. I had my scan - one, two, three. Because I am a physician, I asked if I could read the scan on the spot with the radiologist. I was told that the radiologist, who also was a friend, was reading the scans from the main hospital today, but if I left my number, they would have her call me.

About twenty minutes later as I pulled into the Publix parking lot, my phone rang and the caller ID showed Baptist Hospital. I knew it was my radiologist with the results. I answered, "Hello. What could you see?" It turned out that I had a slightly herniated disc[1] in my lower back which accounted for the pain.

BUT, then came the shocker of my life. "Vince, I also see something suspicious in your left kidney and the way it lights up with the contrast. I hate to say, but I think it's Renal Cell Cancer." My world came to a screeching halt, and time seemed to stand still. I am a doctor. I'm not supposed to get cancer. In fact, I help cure it, so this can't be happening. A million thoughts went racing through my head and then her voice brought me back to reality. "It looks like its about 2.5 centimeters and looks partially cystic[2], but I am pretty sure it's cancer." Again, THAT word!!!!! CANCER. Impossible!! It can't be in ME. I asked her, "Are you sure?" She replied, "I would bet my career on it." She asked me if I knew a good urologist, which I did. She would forward a copy of my films to his office and told me I

1 http://www.webmd.com/back-pain/tc/herniated-disc-topic-overview
2 http://en.wikipedia.org/wiki/Renal_cell_carcinoma

should go see him as soon as possible. I thanked her, still feeling it was all a bad dream.

I sat in my car for what seemed like an hour. My kids. My wife. MY LIFE. "What is going to happen? No, wait, calm down. It may not be a death sentence. Maybe it got caught early and I can beat this thing. Yep, I'll BET I CAN BEAT IT!!! Oh no, what if I can't?" These thoughts kept running through my head. I had seen countless patients with cancer come to the operating room. Some survive their ordeal and some don't. "Which would I be?" Then it really hit me and tears welled up in my eyes.

Cancer, the dreaded "C" word, and it was growing inside of me.

I immediately called my urologist and told his office that I needed to talk to him right away. He was in surgery. I asked where and placed a call to the operating room. I told the nurse that I urgently needed to speak to him. When he answered, I explained everything and asked when he could take this thing out of me. He tried his best to calm me down, and his words helped. "At 2.5 centimeters, you have a great chance of living a long, normal life. The odds change when it reaches 4 centimeters. Then things can be bad. But at 2.5 centimeters, it will be all OK, so calm down. Call my office and come see me this afternoon after I finish surgery." I promptly called the office and made the appointment for 3:00 pm. It was only 12:30 pm. What would I do for the next 2.5 hours? I might go crazy waiting that long.

Suddenly my cellular rang. It was my wife, Maryam, calling to see how the test went. What would I tell her? How can I break the news to her? Is it something to really tell someone over the phone? She will know something is wrong by the tone of my voice, I am sure. I decided to let the call go to voicemail, and I drove home to tell her the news.

When I got home, Maryam instantly knew something was wrong by the look on my face. I told her with tears in my eyes. She sobbed, "Maybe it's a mistake… maybe they need to repeat the scan… maybe another radiologist needs to read it and see if they think the same." "Maryam, it's not necessary. My radiologist is sure of what she saw." We hugged. I explained the urologist was not overly concerned and we had a 3pm appointment. My wife replied, "I'm going with you, no matter what."

It was three o'clock in the waiting room. It seemed like an eternity. "Dr. Conte?" came the call. We both followed the nurse into the exam room. I couldn't sit. I was pacing back and forth in this little room that was no bigger than eight by ten. My friend came in dressed in his white coat with two x-rays in his hands. He smiled, shook my hand, put the films up on the board and flipped on the light. As the lights flashed on, illuminating the x-rays, I immediately focused in on my left kidney. BOOM! There it was, the little wretched alien, the THING growing inside of me. I could see it as plain as day. "Well, here it is," he pointed right to what I was looking at. "In fact, I think it is less than 2.5 centimeters. It measures more like 2 or 1.8 centimeters, which is even better." "So what do I do now?" I asked. "We take it out, do a partial nephrectomy[3], and leave the rest of the kidney behind." Easy for him to say. "When can you do it? Next Monday?" he replied. That was five days away. What if it grew more, or worse – metastasized? "I have to wait five days? I want it out NOW!" He joked about just lying down and operating right here in his office. I wasn't in a joking mood. "OK, next week, Monday." I asked, "What time?" He answered, "7:30 am at Baptist. See my O.R. coordinator and she will set everything up." I needed to get the alien out of me as soon as possible. I began my preoperative journey which would include lab tests, an ECG[4], a CXR[5], and a letter from my cardiologist saying that my blood pressure was under control and it was okay to cut me.

August 5, 2005, could not come soon enough. I slept very little over the next four days, especially Sunday night. "Nothing to eat or drink after midnight" were the specific instructions. I was ready to go. "What if I don't wake up? Or, what if there is a problem and I bleed and need blood and end up in the ICU?" Again, a million thoughts raced in my mind. Finally the alarm went off at 5:30 am. I think I slept two hours total that night.

We both got dressed in silence avoiding the issue. My wife wanted to drive, so I took my packed bag and climbed into the passenger's seat. I kissed my children goodbye as they slept, and I wondered if I would ever see them again. They say that doctors make the worse patients, and I think that is true because we know what can happen and always think that it will happen to us.

We arrived at the hospital and got called into the pre-op area where I changed into my gown, had my IV started, and got some drugs for my severe anxiety. I waited for my surgeon. He finally arrived and as I was being wheeled out, I kissed my wife goodbye and whispered, "I love you." I saw her lips move, but in the noisy room, I was unable to make out what she said.

In the operating room, I was anesthetized without a problem. I woke up in what seemed to be five to ten minutes later. I was in the recovery room, without pain and wearing an oxygen mask. "I MADE IT!!!" I screamed inside my head.

I spent the next ten days in the hospital recovering, but finally went home, and that experience is a whole other story. Let's just say that it opened my eyes to what patients have to go through and changed my perspective on how I practice medicine.

Every six months, my CAT scans keep coming out negative, and my blood tests are stable. So for now it looks like we caught the alien in time and got it all out. Unfortunately, with every new pain or ache, I think the cancer has returned until finally that ache or pain goes away. It is no fun living like this, but many people do.

I was given a second chance, and I have tried to make the best of it. I appreciate the time with my wife and kids more. I appreciate my work and coworkers more. I just appreciate life in general more than before, or as I call it "BC" (Before Cancer). It is unfortunate that sometimes you need a wake up call like that to stop and smell the roses, but with me the lessons learned will not go wasted. I also have a completely new-found empathy for my patients. Who would have guessed that a slight nagging ache in my lower back would make me a better physician, a better father and husband, and a better human being.

Dr. Conte is a Senior Physician with the Miami-Dade County Health Department working in the Department of Epidemiology, Division of Disease Control.

El Médico,
Se Cura a Sí Mismo

Por Dr. Vincent Conte

Todo comenzó como un molestoso dolor en la parte baja de mi espalda que simplemente no se iba. El Advil lo alivió un poco, pero todavía el dolor volvía. Empeoró durante los siguientes dos meses hasta que finalmente yo paré a un neurólogo colega mío en el pasillo del hospital y le comenté sobre él. Me dio una prescripción para un examen de CAT y me indicó que enviara los resultados a su oficina.

El día de mi examen llegó. Era un bello, soleado miércoles. Yo tuve mi examen – uno, dos, tres. En virtud de que soy un médico, yo pedí leer el examen allí mismo con una radióloga. Me indicaron que la radióloga, quien era también una amistad, estaba leyendo los exámenes en el hospital principal hoy, pero que si yo dejaba mi número, ellos le dirían que me llamara.

Unos veinte minutos después mientras entraba al estacionamiento del Publix, mi teléfono sonó y el identificador de llamadas mostró Baptist Hospital. Yo sabía que era mi radióloga con los resultados. Yo respondí, "Hola. ¿Qué pudiste ver?" Resultó que yo tenía una pequeña hernia en un disco[1] en la parte baja de mi espalda, la cual era la causa del dolor.

PERO, luego vino la sorpresa de mi vida. "Vince, yo también veo algo sospechoso en tu riñón izquierdo y la forma como se ilumina con el contraste. No quisiera decirlo, pero creo que es Cáncer de Célula Renal." Mi mundo se paró todo, y pereció haberse congelado. Yo soy un doctor. Se supone que yo no debo padecer de cáncer. De hecho, yo ayudo a curarlo, por lo tanto esto no debe estar ocurriendo. Un millón de pensamientos pasaban por mi cabeza y luego su voz me trajo de nuevo a la realidad. "Parece como que tiene 2.5 centímetros y se ve parcialmente de quiste[2]", pero estoy bastante segura de que

1 http://www.webmd.com/back-pain/tc/herniated-disc-topic-overview
2 http://en.wikipedia.org/wiki/Renal_cell_carcinoma

es cáncer." Otra vez, ¡ESA palabra! ¡Imposible! No puedo ser YO. Le pregunté otra vez, "¿Estas segura?" Ella contestó, "Apostaría toda mi carrera sobre ello." Ella me preguntó si yo conocía un buen urólogo, el cual sí conocía. Ella enviaría una copia de los exámenes a su oficina y me dijo que yo debía verlo lo más antes posible. Le di las gracias, todavía sintiendo que todo era un mal sueño.

Yo me senté en mi carro por lo que pareció una hora. Mis niños. Mi esposa. MI VIDA. "¿Qué va a pasar?" No, espera, cálmate. No tiene por qué ser una sentencia de muerte. Quizás fue agarrado a tiempo y puedo ganarle la batalla. Sí, ¡APUESTO A QUE LE VOY A GANAR LA BATALLA! Oh no, ¿y si no puedo? Esos pensamientos daban vuelta en mi cabeza. Yo he visto innumerables pacientes que vienen con cáncer al quirófano. Algunos sobreviven esa odisea y otros no. "¿Cuál sería yo?" Luego esto de verdad me golpeó y lágrimas llenaron mis ojos.

Cáncer, la temida palabra "C", y estaba creciendo dentro de mí. Yo inmediatamente llamé a mi urólogo y dije a su oficina que tenía que hablar con él en ese momento. Él estaba en una cirugía. Yo pregunté dónde y realicé una llamada al cuarto de operaciones. Le dije a la enfermera que necesitaba hablar urgentemente con él. Cuando él contestó, le expliqué todo y le pregunté cuándo podía sacar esta cosa de mí. Trató de calmarme lo más que pudo, y sus palabras ayudaron. "Con 2.5 centímetros, tienes un gran chance de vivir una vida larga y normal. Las probabilidades cambian cuando alcanza 4 centímetros. En esos casos la cosa puede ser mala. Pero con 2.5 centímetros, todo estará bien, por lo tanto cálmate. Llama a mi oficina y ven a verme esta tarde después que yo termina la cirugía." Prontamente llamé a su oficina y tomé la cita para las 3:00 pm. Era tan solo las 12:30 pm. ¿Qué haría por las próximas 2.5 horas? Me podía volver loco esperando tanto tiempo.

Repentinamente mi celular repicó. Era mi esposa. Maryam, llamando para saber los resultados de los exámenes. ¿Qué le diría? ¿Cómo podía darle la noticia a ella? ¿Es esto algo que debe decirse por teléfono? Ella sabría que algo andaba mal por el tono de mi voz. Decidí dejar que la llamada la atendiera el contestador automático de teléfono, y manejé a la casa para darle la noticia.

Cuando llegué a la casa, Maryam inmediatamente supo que algo andaba mal de mirarme la cara. Se lo dije con lágrimas en mis ojos.

Ella sollozó, "Quizás sea un error... quizás ellos tengan que repetir el examen... quizás otro radiólogo tiene que leerlo y ver si ellos piensan lo mismo."

"Maryam, no es necesario. Mi radióloga está segura de lo que ella vio."

Nos abrazamos. Le expliqué que mi urólogo no estaba muy preocupado y que tenía una cita a las 3:00 pm. Mi esposa respondió, "De cualquier manera, yo voy contigo."

Eran las 3:00 en punto en la sala de espera. Pareció como una eternidad. "¿Dr. Conte?" vino la llamada. Ambos seguimos a la enfermera a la sala de exámenes. No me pude sentar. Estaba caminando de un lado a otro en ese pequeño cuarto que no era más grande de ocho por diez. Mi amigo vino vestido con su bata blanca con dos rayos equis en sus manos. Él sonrió, me dio la mano, y alumbró las fotografías de rayos equis con la luz. Cuando las luces se prendieron, iluminando los exámenes, inmediatamente me enfoqué en mi riñón izquierdo. ¡Boom! Allí estaba, el miserable invasor, la cosa creciendo dentro de mí. Lo pude ver tan claro como el día.

"Bueno, aquí está," él apuntó a lo que yo estaba mirando. "De hecho, creo que tiene menos de 2.5 centímetros. Mide como 2 ó 1.8 centímetros, lo cual es todavía mejor."

"Entonces, ¿Qué hago ahora?" Pregunté.

"Lo sacamos, hacemos una nefrectomía parcial[3], y dejamos el resto del riñón detrás." Era fácil para él decirlo. "¿Cuándo lo podemos hacer? ¿El próximo lunes?" El preguntó.

Eso era cinco días después. ¿Y si crece más, o se pone peor – hace metástasis? "¿Tengo que esperar cinco días? ¡Yo lo quiero sacar AHORA!" El bromeó acerca de acostarme y meramente operarme allí mismo en su oficina. Yo no estaba en humor de chiste. "OK, la próxima semana, el lunes." Yo pregunté, "¿A qué hora?"

"7:30 am en el Baptist. Ve a mi coordinadora de O.R. y ella arreglará todo," contestó.

Yo necesitaba sacar al invasor lo antes posible de mí. Comencé mi viaje preoperatorio lo cual incluía exámenes de laboratorio, un ECG[4], un CXR[5], y una carta de mi cardiólogo diciendo que mi presión sanguínea estaba bajo control y que era okay operarme.

3 http://en.wikipedia.org/wiki/Nephrectomy
4 http://en.wikipedia.org/wiki/Ecg
5 http://www.enotes.com/surgery-encyclopedia/chest-x-ray

El 5 de agosto del 2005, no pudo venir lo suficientemente rápido. Yo dormí muy poco durante los siguientes cuatro días, especialmente el domingo en la noche. "Nada de comer o tomar después de medianoche" fueron las instrucciones específicas. Estaba listo para irme. "¿Y si no me despierto? O, ¿Y si tengo un problema y me desangro y necesito sangre y termino en el ICU?" Otra vez, un millón de pensamientos corrían en mi mente. Finalmente la alarma sonó a las 5:30 am. Creo que dormí dos horas en total esa noche.

Ambos nos vestimos en silencio. Mi esposa quiso manejar, por lo que yo agarré mi maletín y me monté en la silla del pasajero. Me despedí de mis hijos besándolos mientras dormían, y me pregunté si alguna vez los volvería a ver. Se dice que los doctores son los peores pacientes, y creo que es verdad porque sabemos lo que puede pasar y siempre pensamos que nos va a pasar.

Llegamos al hospital y nos llamaron al área de preoperatorio donde yo me puse mi bata, me pusieron mi IV, y me dieron medicinas para mi ansiedad severa. Esperé por mi cirujano. Finalmente llegó y mientras me llevaban en silla de rueda, le di un beso de despedida a mi esposa y le susurré, "Te quiero." Yo le vi sus labios mover, pero con el ruido que había en el cuarto, no pude descifrar lo que quiso decir.

En el cuarto de operaciones, fui anestesiado sin problemas. Me desperté en lo que pareció de cinco a diez minutos después. Estaba en la sala de recuperación, sin dolor y utilizando una máscara de oxigeno. "!!!LO LOGRE!!!" Grité dentro de mi cabeza.

Estuve los siguientes diez días en el hospital recuperándome, pero finalmente fui a casa, y esa experiencia es otra historia completa. Déjenme tan solo decirles que abrió mis ojos a lo que los pacientes tienen que pasar y cambió mi perspectiva de cómo yo practico la medicina.

Cada seis meses, mis exámenes de CAT siguen resultando negativos, y mis exámenes de sangre son estables. Por ahora parece que capturamos el invasor a tiempo y lo sacamos completo. Desgraciadamente, con cada dolor o malestar pienso que el cáncer a retornado hasta que finalmente ese dolor o molestia se va.

Me fue dado un segundo chance, y he tratado de sacar lo mejor de él. Aprecio más el tiempo con mi esposa e hijos. Aprecio más mi trabajo y compañeros de trabajo. Simplemente aprecio la vida más que antes, o como yo lo llamo "BC" (Antes del Cáncer). Es desafortunado que algunas veces tú necesitas una llamada que te despierte como esa a fin de parar y oler las flores, pero conmigo las lecciones aprendidas no serán desperdiciadas. Yo también he encontrado una completamente nueva empatía por mis pacientes. Quién hubiese adivinado que un leve molestoso dolor en la parte baja de mi espalda me habría hecho un mejor médico, mejor padre y esposo, y un mejor ser humano. ☼

Dr. Conte es un Médico Superior del Departamento de Salud del Condado de Miami-Dade trabajando para el Departamento de Epidemiología, División de Control de Enfermedad.

Doktè geri tèt ou ou menm

Po Dr. Vincent Conte

Maladi a te kòmanse tankou yon ti mal do ki te ap zigonnen mwen anba rèl do mwen, epi ki te derefize sispan. Lè mwen te bwè Advil doulè a te pase men li pate disparèt. Doulè a te vinn pi mal nan de mwa ki te finn pase yo jouktan yon jou nan koulwa lopital la mwen rete yon konfrè mwen , yon doktè ki okipe maladi nè epi mwen di li zafè maladi mwen a. Li ban mwen yon preskripsyon pou mwen ale fè yon egzamen CAT scan (tès ki tankou yon radyografi ki montre foto pati nan kò yon moun nan tout pozisyon) epi li di mwen pou mwen voye rezilta yo nan klinik li.

Jou a te vini pou mwen te al fè tès CAT scan la . Se te yon jou plen solèy nan yon Mèkredi lè mwen te fè tès la trap de, en , de , twa. Paske mwen se yon doktè mwen te mande eske mwen te kapab li tès la tou swit ansanb ak doktè espesyalist radyografi a. Yo te di mwen ke dokte radyologist la ki se yon zanmi mwen tap li rezilta tès Cat scan yo nan lopital la jou sa a. Epi ke si mwen te kite nimewo telefòn mwen li ta va rele mwen. Apre ven minit pandan mwen tap antre nan paking sipèmakèt yo rele Publix la, telefòn mwen te sonnen epi pati ki make nimewo moun ki ap rele a te make ke se te lopital Baptist . Mwen te konnen ke se te doktè radyologi a ki tap rele ak rezilta tès yo . Mwen reponn : »alo ki sa ke ou te kapab wè ». Sa ki te pase se ke mwen te genyen yon zo nan kolon vètebral mwen ki te deplase an ba nan rèl do mwen se sa ki te fè ke mwen te genyen doulè a.

Men lè sa a bagay ki te ban mwen pi gwo sezisman nan lavi mwen te rive. Doktè radyologi a di mwen »Vince mwen wè yon bagay ki kapab yon maladi grav nan ren gòch ou epi jan ke ren gòch la klere lè yo mete aparèy sou li mwen rayi pou mwen di ou sa mwen pral di ou a men mwen kwè ke se yon kansè ki la nan selil nan ren ou yo. La vi mwen rete bip, epi se te kòm si tan a te rete bloke depi lè sa a. Mwen se yon doktè mwen pa sipoze gen kansè. Epi tout okontrè mwen ede trete kansè sa pa fouti ap rive mwen. Genyen yon milyon lide ki pase nan tèt mwen epi se vwa doktè radyografi a ki fè mwen tounen nan realite sa ki te ap pase a. Li te di mwen : » Li sanble ke kansè a gen 2.5 santimèt epi li sanble ke gen yon pati ki se yon kist. Men mwen pi si ke se kansè ». Pawòl kansè sa a ankò , se pa posib, li pa kapab lakay mwen . Mwen mande li eske li te si de sa ke li te ap di a. Li reponn mwen : »map parye sou sa mwen di a. »Li mande mwen si mwen te konnen yon bon doktè ki okipe maladi nan ren doktè yo rele irolojist yo. Mwen te konnen yon doktè irolojist. Doktè radyografi a te di mwen ke li ta pral voye yon foto radyografi yo bay doktè irolojist la epi ke mwen te dwe al wè doktè irolojist la tou swit pi vit ke mwen te kapab. Mwen di doktè a mesi men mwen te santi ke tout bagay sa a se te yon rèv. Mwen chita nan otomobil mwen pandan sa ki te sanble yon è de tan. Piti mwen yo, madanm mwen, lavi mwen . Sak pral pase mwen ? Non tann, kalme ou. Li kapab pa vle di se yon santans lanmò. Petèt kòm yo jwen li bonè mwen kapab pote la viktwa sou bagay sa a. O ! non e si kansè a ta va mete do mwen atè. Tout lide sa yo tap kouri nan tèt mwen, Mwen te wè tèlman pasyan, moun malad ak kansè pase sou tab operasyon. Genyen ki te pote la viktwa genyen ki te pèdi batay la. Kilès nan yo ke mwen ta pral ye ? Lè sa a bagay la pote mwen nan tèt epi dlo tonbe koule nan je mwen. Kansè maladi ki an anglè komanse ak lèt C a ki mete laperèz nan kò tout moun la, epi bagay si la te ap pouse andedan mwen. Menm moman mwen rele klinik doktè irolojist mwen a epi mwen di li ke mwen te bezwen pale ak li tou swit. Doktè irolojist la te ap fè operasyon li te okipe. Mwen mande nan kilès lopital li te ap fè operasyon yo epi mwen rele li nan telefòn lopital la. Mwen di enfimyè a ki te reponn la ke mwen te bezwen pale ak doktè a tou swit. Lè doktè a reponn, mwen esplike li tout bagay epi mwen mande li ki lè ke li te kapab retire timè sa a nan kò mwen. Li eseye jan ke li te kapab pou li te kalme mwen epi pawòl li yo te ede mwen. Li di mwen ak yon timè ki 2 santimèt 5 ou genyen anpil chans pou ou viv lontan yon lavi ki nòmal. Se lè kansè a mezire 4 santimèt ke li kapab move. Men lè ke se 2.5 santimèt tout bagay ap nan plas yo. Kidonk kalme ou. Rele klinik mwen a epi vini wè mwen apremidi a lè mwen fini travay nan sal operasyon. Byen vit mwen rele klinik doktè a epi mwen pran yon randevou pou twa zè an apremidi. Li te midi trant sèlman lè ke mwen te rele a , sa mwen te dwe fè pandan 2 è edmi de tan? Tèt mwen ta kapab pati nan tann tout tan sa a. Menm moman a telefòn selilè mwen te sonnen. Se te madanm mwen ki te bezwen konnen ki jan tès yo te pase. Sa mwen dwe di li ?Ki jan pou mwen fè pou mwen ba li move nouvèl sa a ? Eske se yon kalite nouvèl yon moun kapab bay nan telefòn ? Si mwen te pale li te ap konnen ke gen yon bagay ki pa nan plas li lè li tande son vwa mwen. Mwen deside pou mwen kite aparèy telefòn la pran apèl la epi mwen deside kondwi otomobil mwen pou mwen ba li nouvèl la lè mwen rive lakay mwen. Lè mwen rive lakay mwen Maryam te konnen menm moman a ke te gen yon bagay dwòl ki te ap pase lè li gade figi mwen. Ak dlo nan je, mwen rakonte li sa ki te ap ap pase mwen. Li tap krye tou. Petèt se te yon erè ? petèt yo te dwe refè tès yo? petèt yon lòt doktè radyografi ta dwe li radyografi yo pou wè si li menm tou wè bagay yo menm jan Maryam te ap di mwen. Mwen di li Maryam se pa nesesè pou nou fè tout sa, dokte ki li radyolgrafi mwen yo di ke li si tankou zo janb pè etènèl de sa ke li wè a. Nou anbrase, li pase men li nan kou mwen mwen pase men mwen nan kou li epi mwen esplike li ke doktè irolojist la te kwè ke paske kansè a te piti ka a pa te twò grav epi ke mwen te gen randevou ak epesyalist la a 3 è. Madanm mwen te reponn mwen : »mwen prale ak ou nan randevou a, nenpòt ki jan.

Li te twa zè nan sal atant klinik la, li te sanble ke yon etènite te pase . Yo rele mwen pou mwen antre nan konsiltasyon, mwen menm ak madanm mwen swiv enfimyè a nan sal konsiltasyon a. Mwen pa te kapab chita mwen te ap ale vini nan ti pyès la ki te mezire yuit pa dis. Zanmi doktè mwen a vini ak blouz blanch long li sou li epi ak de radyografi nan men li. Li souri, li ban mwen lanmen epi li mete radyografi yo sou bwat ki gen limyè yo sèvi pou li radyografi yo. Li limen limyè a sou radyografi yo. Menm moman a mwen brake je mwen sou kote ren gòch la te parèt sou radyografi a. WOY ! li te la menm , ti malveant etranje a , bagay la ki te ap donnen andedan mwen a. Mwen te kapab wè li klè tankou moun wè byen lè li fè klè .

« Ebyen men li » li pwente dwèt li sou sa ke mwen te ap gade a. Mwen byen kwè tou ke reèlman vre li pi piti ke 2.5 santimèt. Li mezire apeprè 2 oswa 1.8 santimèt sa ki fè ke mwen genyen yon pi bon chans toujou pou mwen sove. « Kidonk sa mwen dwe fè kounye a » ? mwen mande. Nap retire li nou ap fè yon operasyon pou retire yon pati nan ren a sa yo rele nefrektomi epi nou ap kite rès ren a

deyè kote li ye a. Se te fasil pou li di mwen sa. «Kilè ou kapab fè li» ?
Eske lendi pwochen ap bon pou ou li mande mwen. Se te nan senk
jou. E si pandan tan sa a li pouse pi gwo oswa sa ki pi mal si li gaye
voye pitit nan lòt pati nan kò mwen? Kouman se pou mwen tann
senk jou? Mwen mande li.» Mwen vle ou retire li KOUNYE a «mwen
di li, Li fè yon blag ak mwen epi li di mwen ebyen nou kapab tou
opere ou la menm nan klinik la sou tab konsiltasyon a. Mwen pa te
sou fè blag. «Dakò lendi pwochen» mwen di li. A ki lè mwen mande
li. «Set è trant di maten nan Baptist. Wè ak moun ki okipe zafè
ka operasyon mwen yo epi li va ranje tout bagay pou ou «li reponn
mwen. Mwen te bezwen retire bagay etranje sa a nan kò mwen pi
vit ki te posib. Mwen te kòmanse prepare mwen pou operasyon a ak
yon kantite demach nan fè egzamen laboratwa, nan fè egzamen pou
kè ak egzamen kòf lestomak mwen pou tcheke poumon ak kè mwen.
Ak yon lèt ki soti nan men doktè espesyalist kè ki di ke tansyon,
mwen te bon epi ke yo te kapab opere mwen san ke kè mwen ta va
bay pwoblèm.

Mwen pa te kapab tann pou jou ki te 5 daout, 2005 la te rive.
Mwen pa te preske domi ditou pandan kat jou ki te pase yo sitou
dimanch swa. Yo te byen eksplike mwen pou mwen pa te bwè ak
manje anyen apre minwi. Men te pare pou mwen te ale. E si mwen
pa te leve nan operasyon a? E si te genyen yon pwoblèm epi mwen
te senyen twòp epi mwen te bezwen san epi mwen te vin ateri nan
sal swen entansif ? Epi, epi yon milyon lide te ap kouri galope nan
tèt mwen, alafen dè fen revèy la sonnen a senk è trant dimaten.
Mwen kwè ke mwen domi selman 2 è de tan an tout nan nwit sa a.
Madanm mwen ak mwen, nou tou le de mete rad sou nou san pale,
nou te ap evite pale sou koze maladi mwen a. Madanm mwen te
vle kondwi otomobil la, kidonk mwen pran malèt mwen epi mwen
monte nan plas pasaje a. Mwen te bo ti moun yo pandan ke yo te ap
domi mwen te ap mande tèt mwen si mwen te ap janm wè yo anko.
Yo toujou di ke doktè se pi move patyan e mwen kwè ke se vre paske
nou menm doktè konnen byen sa ki kapab rive epi nou toujou kwè ke
move bagay sa yo ap rive nou.

Nou te rive lopital la epi yo te rele mwen nan kote yo pare moun
pou al nan operayon a. Nan kote sa a mwen retire rad mwen pou
mwen mete kimono moun ki pral opere yo. Yo te mete yon seròm
pou mwen epi yo te ban mwen medikaman pou anpeche mwen gen

kè sote. Mwen te tann doktè chirijyen mwen a. Li te fini pa rive epi yo te roule mwen sou charyo a. Mwen te bo madanm mwen pou di li orevwa epi mwen te di li : » mwen renmen ou ». Mwen wè madanm mwen bat boucch li men te gen twòp bwi nan sal la pou mwen te tande sa li te di mwen.

Nan sal operasyon a mwen te pran anestezi a san okenn pwoblèm. Mwen te leve nan sa ki te sanble senk a dis minit apre yo te andomi mwen a. Mwen te nan sal pou moun leve apre operasyon a mwen pa te genyen doulè epi mwen te genyen yon mask oxijèn nan figi mwen. « MWEN CHAPE » mwen te rele byen fò andedan tèt mwen.

Mwen pase di jou nan lopital la pou mwen te refè epi mwen te fini pa ale lakay mwen. Eksperyans sa a se te yon lòt istwa. An nou di sèlman ke sa mwen te pase a te louvri je mwen pou mwen wè sa patyan yo ap pase lè yo gen yon maladi epi sa fè ke mwen chanje anpil jan ke mwen fè metye doktè a.

Chak sis mwa tès CAT scan mwen yo kontinye vinn jwen mwen san pwoblèm maladi nan yo, epi tès san mwen yo bon tou. Kidonk pou kounye a li sanble ke nou te trape byen bonè kansè a, vye bagay etranje ki te ap donnen nan kò mwen a, epi nou te retire li nèt. Malerezman chak fwa ke mwen gen yon ti doulè, yon ti ko fè mal, mwen mete nan tèt mwen ke kansè a retounen lide sa rete nan tèt mwen jouktan doulè a oswa kò fè mal la disparèt nèt. Mwen pa genyen kè kontan lè mwen ap viv ak kè sote konsa, men gen anpil moun ki ap viv konsa.

Mwen te jwen yon dezyèm chans nan lavi a se pou mwen te sèvi ak li byen. Mwen apresye plis tan mwen gen pou mwen pase ak madanm mwen epi ak pitit mwen yo. Mwen apresye travay mwen ak kanmarad travay mwen plis. Mwen apresye lavi an jeneral pi plis kounye a ke avan maladi a te antre sou mwen,oswa jan mwen rele li «B.C.» B a se pou avan an anglè C a se pou kansè ki ekri ak yon C an anglè, B.C. vle di avan kansè. Malerezman anpil fwa yon moun bezwen pase yon move ka dè konsa pou li souke kò li epi aprann gade bagay nan lavi a yon lòt jan. Tankou yo di pran yon ti tan pou chèche yon flè ròz epi santi li pou respire pafen li. Nan ka pa mwen leson ke mwen aprann la pap gaspiye. Mwen remake ke kounye a mwen gen

pi bon kè nan travay mwen ak moun malad. Ki moun ki ta kwè ke
yon ti doulè ki te ap manje mwen nan rèl do mwen ta kab fè mwen
vini yon pi bon doktè, yon pi bon papa, yon pi bon mari, epi yon pi
bon moun tou. ☼

*Doktè Comte se yon doktè wo grade nan pami doktè yo ki ap travay
nan depatman sante piblik nan Miami nan biwo ki okipe epidemi ak
kontwòl maladi.*

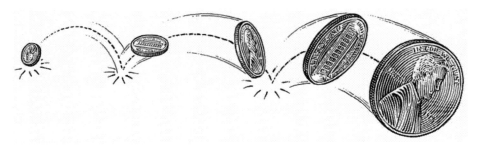

The Collector

By Mort Laitner

As I opened the door of my SUV, I glanced down at the ground and observed a worn penny. My spirits lifted. Had I found a valuable coin to add to my numismatic past? I observed Lincoln's presidential face, the year 1941 and the mint mark "D." Since its Denver creation, sixty-seven years ago, this coin had made it to Miami. I automatically flipped the coin over.

The copper cent was also known as a wheat penny from the design on its back.

As I flipped the coin, my mind flashed back to the Colonial Inn Motel (181 Street and Collins, Miami Beach). Who can forget the white marbled horses pulling a freshly painted black four-wheel buggy, complete with cement steps for the tourists to climb aboard. What a photo op! The year was 1959 and a ten-year-old coin collector studied the mound of change his father had deposited on the motel writing desk.

The boy found a 1909 VDB Lincoln penny in this mound. Over the next eight years, he collects Franklin halves, Morgan dollars, Indian head cents… Coin collecting was more than a hobby, it was a mild obsession and he treasured his coins as much as his first girlfriend, his '67 Mustang or his Head skis.

As I inserted the penny into my wallet for safekeeping, I noticed my Health Department business cards. I began to think about my career. Had I collected any treasures along the way?

First, interesting job titles: the swimming pool solicitor (environmental health), the raccoon attorney (rabies), the laser-beam lawyer (environmental safety), the birdman barrister (psittacosis – parrot fever), and the peepshow prosecutor (AIDS).

Where else but in a Health Department could have I collected these comical monikers?

Then my mind wandered to my days of seeking fame and I realized I had a media collection: CBS National News, New York Times, St. Louis Dispatch, Life and Money magazines.

Where else could a minor league attorney get this national media coverage?
As I scratched my head, I thought of the different hats I have worn with the agency: prosecuted cases, defended cases, and I've even worn the hat of a judge. I've drafted legislation.

Where else but a Health Department?
I wear many others hats: building project manager, film director, producer and a bio-terrorism field exercise coordinator, party planner, author and lecturer. And now, I am writing and publishing. Where else but in the Health Department could I have the freedom to venture out into so many fields?

Next, I thought about my collection of interesting experiences:
The experience of saving a newborn's life (obtaining a court-ordered blood transfusion);

- Being cursed by a gypsy in an adoption case (so far the curse hasn't taken hold, wait a minute... my weight gain...the patch);
- Having my life threatened by a young man, (whose water well we determined was contaminated.) He angrily had yelled over the phone, "I got a bullet in my gun with your name on it." Without fear, I calmly gave him a wrong address;
- The AIDS related case in the Key West, (where from the moment I got on the plane in Miami, people were talking about the case, and the general hum of gossip continued at the Key West Airport, during my Taxi ride to the hotel and my walk down Duval street on the way to the Courthouse.) The whole town was abuzz with my case.

Where else but the Health Department?
I've even collected a number of memorable character witnesses:
- Sir Lancelot Jones[1], a well-read gentle man who taught US presidents how to bone fish in the Keys;
- A soldier who dropped the A-bomb on Nagasaki;
- Rudolf Hess' US army doctor at Spandau prison;
- Evil Eye Finkle[2], who used his looks to intimidate boxers at ringside.

Where else but the Health Department could I meet these interesting individuals?
At lunch, I opened my wallet to pay for my meal. The penny jumped out and hit the ground. Heads! As I picked up the coin, I observed the President's face, Abe smiled: "Son, You're lucky you chose a career in public health."

1 http://atlanta.creativeloafing.com/gyrobase/Content?oid=oid%3A11049
2 http://www.thesweetscience.com/boxing-article/2245/evil-eye-finkle-two-parts-voodoo-one-part-fraud

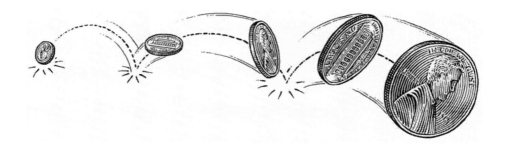

El Coleccionista

Por Mort Laitner

ientras habría la puerta de mi SUV, miré hacia abajo rápidamente y observé un centavo desgastado. Mi espíritu se levantó. ¿Habré encontrado una moneda de valor a fin de añadirla a mi numismático pasado? Observé la cara del Presidente Lincoln, el año 1941 y la marca de emisión "D". Como es una creación de Denver, sesenta y siete años atrás, esta moneda logró llegar a Miami. Yo inmediatamente volteé la moneda.

El centavo de cobre también era conocido como un centavo de trigo por el diseño de su dorso.

Mientras volteaba la moneda mi mente se remontó al Motel Colonial Inn (Calle 181 y Collins, Miami Beach). Quién puede olvidar los caballos de mármol blanco empujando un cochecito negro de cuatro ruedas de pintura fresca, completado con escaleras de cemento para los turistas montarse. ¡Que foto! Era el año 1959 y un coleccionista de diez años estudió la pila de cambio que su padre había depositado en el escritorio del motel.

El niño encontró un centavo de Lincoln VDB de 1909 en esta pila. Durante los siguientes ocho años, él coleccionaba medio dólares de Franklin, dólares de Morgan, centavos de cabeza de indios... El coleccionar monedas era más que un hobby, era una obsesión menor y él apreciaba a sus monedas tanto como a su primera novia, su Mustang del '67 o sus esquís Head.

Mientras insertaba el centavo en mi cartera para guardarlo, noté mis tarjetas de presentación del Departamento de Salud. Comencé a pensar en mi carrera. ¿He colectado algunos tesoros en el camino?

Primero, títulos de trabajo interesantes: el abogado de piscinas (salud ambiental), el abogado mapache (rabias), el abogado rayo-láser (salvaguarda ambiental), el abogado hombre pájaro (psitacosis – fiebre de pájaro), y abogado acusador de casas de entretenimiento (SIDA).

¿En dónde más que en el Departamento de Salud pude haber colectado estos nombres cómicos? Luego mi mente se remontó a mis días de buscar fama y me di cuenta que tenía una colección de medios de comunicación: CBS National News, New York Times, St. Louis Dispatch, Life Money magazines.

¿En dónde más un abogado de pequeñas ligas logra esta cobertura nacional en los medios de comunicación? Mientras me rascaba la cabeza, pensé en los diferentes sombreros que yo he usado en la agencia: abogado acusador y defensor, redacté leyes y he también utilizado el sombrero de juez.

¿En dónde más que en el Departamento de Salud? Yo he utilizado muchos otros sombreros: manager de proyecto de construcción, director de película, productor y coordinador de ejercicios de campo de bio-terrorismo, organizador de fiestas, autor y orador. Y ahora, estoy escribiendo y publicando.

¿En dónde más que en el Departamento de Salud pude haber yo tenido la libertad de aventurarme hacia tantos campos? Luego, pensé en mi colección de diferentes experiencias:
- La experiencia de salvar la vida de un recién nacido (obteniendo una orden de la corte para transfusión de sangre);
- El ser maldecido por un gitano en un caso de adopción (hasta ahora la maldición no se ha cumplido, espera un momento... mi subida de peso... mi parche);
- El ser amenazada mi vida por un hombre joven, (cuyo pozo de agua nosotros determinamos estaba contaminado.) Él gritó bravamente por el teléfono, "Tengo una bala en mi pistola con tu nombre sobre ella." Sin miedo, calmadamente le di a él una dirección equivocada;

- El caso relacionado al SIDA en Key West, (donde desde el momento que me monté en el avión en Miami, la gente estaba hablando sobre el caso, y el murmullo general del chisme continuó en el Aeropuerto de Key West, durante mi recorrido en el taxi al hotel y en mi camino a la calle Duval en la vía al edificio de tribunales). El pueblo entero estaba murmurando sobre mi caso.

¿En dónde más que en el Departamento de Salud? Yo hasta he coleccionado un número de memorables testigos de reputación:
- Sir Lancelot Jones1, un caballero bien leído que ha enseñado a presidentes de USA como pescar con hueso en los Keys;
- Un soldado que lanzó la bomba atómica en Nagazaki;
- El doctor de la Armada de USA Rudolph Hess en la prisión de Spandau;
- Evil Eye Finkle7, quien utilizó su apariencia para intimidar boxeadores en el ring.

¿En dónde más que en el Departamento de Salud pude haber conocido estos individuos interesantes? En el almuerzo, abrí mi cartera para pagar por mi comida. El centavo saltó y se cayó al suelo. ¡Cara! Mientras recogía la moneda, observé la cara del Presidente, Abe sonrió: "Hijo, tienes suerte de haber escogido una carrera en salud pública."

---

1 http://atlanta.creativeloafing.com/gyrobase/Content?oid=oid%3A11049
2 http://www.thesweetscience.com/boxing-article/2245/evil-eye-finkle-two-parts-voodoo-one-part-fraud

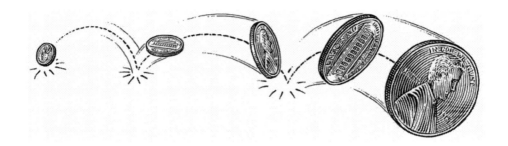

Moun ki
ap fè koleksyon

By Mort Laitner

Pandan mwen ap louvri pòt otomobil jip mwen a, mwen gade atè a epi mwen wè yon senk kòb penich ki te finn depatcha. Kè mwen te kontan. Eske se te yon lajan ra ke mwen tap kapab ajoute nan koleksyon mwen te konnen fè a a? Mwen gade foto Prezidan Lincoln ak lane 1941 ki te grave sou sou kòb la epi lèt D ki te make sou li kòm mak fabrik li. Depi gen a peprè 67 lane ke lajan sa a te fabrike nan vil Denver, kounye a li i vinn ateri jouk nan Miami. Sanzatann mwen te vire pyès lajan a.

Lajan kwiv la yo te rele li tou ble akòz de desen zepi ble ki te nan do li a.

Pandan ke mwen ap vire pyès lajan sou lòt bò li a, lide mwen ale sou yon motèl nan Miami yo rele Colonial Inn Motel ki nan adrès 181 ak Collins nan Miami Beach. Ki moun ki kapab blye chwal blan ki te ap rale yon bogi yo fèk pentire an nwa epi ki te genyen kat wou, li te konplèt ak mach an siman pou touris yo te kapab monte andedan bogi a? Ala yon bon chans li te ye pou moun pwofite fè foto! Se te lane 1959 epi yon ti moun dizan ki te ap fè koleksyon pyès lajan tap gade pakèt pil lajan an pyès ke papa li te depoze sou biwo pou moun ekri nan lotèl la.

Ti gason a te genyen yon senk kòb penich Lincoln VDB nan pil la. Nan yuitan apre sa li te ap fè koleksyon mwatye dola ak foto Franklin sou yo. Dola ak foto Morgan sou yo, pyès santim ak tèt endyen sou yo. ....Zafè Koleksyon pyès lajan sila a se pa te yon distraksyon sèlman se te yon obsesyon epi jenn nonm la te renmen pyès lajan li yo otan ke premye menaj li, Mustang 67 li a, ak bagay li sèvi pou li fè ski yo.

Pandan ke mwen te ap sere senk kòb penich la nan bous mwen pou li pa te pèdi, mwen wè kat biznis mwen kòm anplwaye depatman sante piblik la. Mwen komanse sonje ki jan karyè mwen te ye. Eske mwen te ranmase okenn trezò pandan ke mwen te ap fè karyè mwen nan depatman lasante a.

Tou dabò se te tit travay mwen yo ki ta kab fè ke yon moun ta renmen yo epi vle fè koleksyon ak yo : « Moun ki ap mache mande pou pisin yo », (nan lasante anviwònman) «avoka bèt raccon » (maladi laraj), «avoka ki ap voye limyè sou zafè lasante anviwònman », «avoka zwazo» (maladi psittakòz, ak paròt fever) avoka prosekitè ki ap rapouswiv moun ki ap fè demonstrasyon ak pati prive kò yo (maladi Sida).

Ki lòt kote ke nan depatman sante piblik mwen ta va koleksyonen tout ti non jwèt komik sa yo? Epi lespri mwen ale flannen sou epòk mwen tap chèche renome epi mwen realize ke mwen te genyen tou yon koleksyon rankont ak jounalist tankou CBS, Nation News, New-York Times, St Louis Dispatch, Life ak Money Magazines.

Ki lòt kote ke yon avoka ki pa te nan gwoup gran nèg peyi a te kapab fè pale de li konsa nan medya, radyo, joual, televizyon tout peyi a? pandan mwen te ap grate tèt mwen, mwen sonje tout kalite chapo ke mwen te mete sa vle di tout kalite travay ke mwen te fè pandan mwen tap travay nan ajans sa a : mwen te travay kòm avoka ki ap rapouswiv moun nan ka nan lajistis, epi kom avoka ki te defann lwa ki te pral la chamb pou yo vote yo, mwen te menm fè yon kout jij tou.

Kilès kote ke nan depatman lasante? Mwen te mete divès chapo pou mwen te fè divès travay, mwen te manadje pwojè konstriksyon nan depatman a, mwen te fè direktè film sinema tou, pwodiktè film sinema tou. Koodinatè ki te okipe zafè repetityon sou teren pou lite kont teworist ak pwodwi vivan. Moun ki ap oganize fèt, ekriven epi moun ki ap fè konferans, epi kounye a mwen ap ekri ak piblye liv tou.

Kilès lòt kote ke nan depatman lasante mwen tap jwen libète pou mwen tounen yon touch a tou nan tout kalite metye? Mwen sonje koleksyon eksperyans enteresan yo.

- Eksperyans pou sove lavi yon ti bebe ki fèk fèt (lè mwen te genyen pwose pou la jistis bay lòd pou bay timoun nan san li te bezwen.
- Lè ke yon gipsi te ba mwen madichon nan yon ka adopsyon (Jouk kounye a madichon an pa pran sou mwen, tann yon minit jan mwen vinn two gwo a, epi patch map sèvi pou mwen sispan fimen ou kwè ke se pa madichon?)
- Jan ke yon jenn gason menase lavi mwen (Lè ke nou te deklare ke pyi dlo li a te te genyen jem maladi ladan li.) Li te move anpil nan telefòn nan lè li te rele:» mwen gen yon bal nan revolvè mwen ak non ou make sou li». San okenn lapèrez nan kò mwen mwen te bali yon move adrès.
- Ka nan Key West ki te gen pou wè ak maladi Sida) kote ke moun tap pale de ka sa a depi mwen monte avyon sot Miami pou mwen ale Key West epi gwondman tripotaj sou ka a te kontinye nan aeropò Key West la pandan mwen te monte taxi a pou mwen ale nan lotèl la epi tou lè mwen te ap mache nan ri Duval pou mwen ale nan tribinal lajistis la. Tout lavil la te ap boudonnen tankou yon nich gèp.

Ki lòt kote ke nan depatman sante piblik? Mwen ta kab fè koleksyon yon kantite temwen gwo zouzoune tankou:

- Sir Lancelot Jones[1] yon ekriven anpil moun li liv li ekri yo epi ki te montre prèzidan lèzetazini kijan pou li te peche pwason yo rele bonefish la nan Key West
- Yon nan milite ki te lage bonb atomik la nan Nagazaki nan peyi Japon
- Rudolf Hess yon moun ki te doktè lame ameriken nan prizon Spandau.
- Evil Eye Finkle[2], yon nom ki te yon move je e ki te sèvi ak figi di li a pou li fè boxsè yo pè lè yo te nan kote yo ap fè match bòx yo.

---

1 http://atlanta.creativeloafing.com/gyrobase/Content?oid=oid%3A11049
2 http://www.thesweetscience.com/boxing-article/2245/evil-eye-finkle-two-parts-voodoo-one-part-fraud

Kilès kote ke nan depatman lasante mwen tap janm kapab rankontre moun enpotan, gwo zouzoun sa yo? Pandan mwen ale manje manje midi mwen mwen louvri bous mwen pou mwen peye manje a , senk kòb penich la soti nan bous mwen, li tombe atè. Li tonbe sou bò ki gen foto tèt tonton a sou li a. Lè mwen ap ranmase pyès lajan a mwen gade figi prezidan Abe (prezidan Lincoln) li souri kòm si li te di» pitit gason ou se yon nonm ki gen chans ou te chwazi yon karyè nan zafè sante pibik.

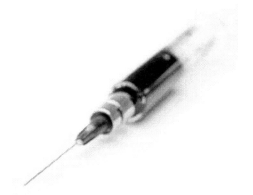

Injected with Fear

By Amy Tejirian

The warm, sunny February day in Los Angeles was the complete antithesis of where I was the day before. I could not believe how hot it was for a winter's day. That morning I had taken a one-way plane ride to LA from Calgary, Canada, the only home I had known in my eleven years. As the plane was taking off, my eyes gushed with tears. I did not want to move. I loved my hometown.

After my family and I had arrived at LAX, my parents immediately tried to enroll me at my new school. The school board informed us that my sister and I needed to get TB tests. My family trekked to the Glendale Health Center a couple blocks away from my new house. As we waited for our turn, I started to feel the fatigue setting in of moving to a new country that morning. Finally, they called my number. I sat down in front of the nurse, and my mom handed her my Canadian immunization record. The nurse glanced at my name then started to ask me questions in some language that was not English. I just stared at her blankly. Then in English she asked, "You are Armenian right?" I nodded. She continued, "You don't speak the language?" I said I did but had no idea that she was speaking Armenian to me. This was a culture shock. In Calgary, when people asked what nationality I was, I responded Armenian.

They would usually look confused and say, "Oh Romanian?" And in Calgary, when I spoke Armenian with my family, it was like our own secret language that no one else could understand. Here in Glendale, most of the city's residents as well as the nursing staff at this Health Department were Armenian, but I could not understand a single word this nurse was saying to me. The nurse decided to speak English. Later, I found out that she was speaking another dialect of Armenian.

The nurse then looked at my immunization record and declared, "Canadians don't know anything about immunizations!" This really offended me. I had just gotten the Rubella vaccine two days earlier in Calgary so that I would be compliant with all of my vaccines. The nurse pulled out a series of needles. She started preparing to give me shots in the arm. I did not understand what she was doing to me. She stabbed me in the arm with one needle, the tetanus shot. She pricked me again with another shot. And finally, she administered the TB injection. It all happened too quickly. I stood up and walked over to my mother to wait for my sister's turn. My sister sat in the same torture chair I had just sat in. All of a sudden I felt woozy. I opened my mouth to explain this to my mother, but as soon as I did, my head started to spin. The next thing I can remember was waking up, lying on an exam table with my feet in the air. The odor of pungent smelling salts irritated my nose. "What happened?" It turns out that I had a little seizure and I fainted. Welcome to America. For the next couple days my arm was incredibly sore from the tetanus shot. I could barely lift it up. After the TB test results came in negative I was allowed to attend school.

Fast forward sixteen years to when I was due to receive another tetanus shot, I avoided it like the plague. I knew it was important to get but my past experience left a bitter taste in my mouth. I could not avoid the tetanus shot forever.

In 2006, the Miami-Dade County Health Department was conducting their employee immunization drive. I wanted to get my flu shot so I had obtained my old immunization record from my high school. I waited as colleague after colleague received vaccines and flu shots. Then it was my turn. I sat in the dreaded chair and handed over my records. It was clear that I was long overdue for my tetanus shot. I was a nervous wreck. The fear ran rampant through my rigid body. Everyone from SIP (Special Immunization Project) was trying to calm me. Tracie, my co-worker, tried to distract me as my arm was getting prepped for the shots. To my surprise, in a couple of minutes it was all over. I didn't feel sick at all. Further, my arm was not sore afterwards.

First Lady Eleanor Roosevelt said it best, "You gain strength, courage and confidence by every experience in which you really stop to look fear in the face. You must do the thing you think you cannot do." That hot, humid Miami afternoon, I looked fear in the face and gained self-confidence. ☼

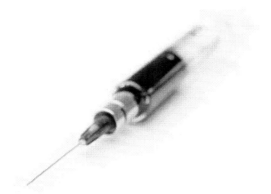

Inyectada con Miedos

Por Amy Tejirian

El caliente, soleado día de febrero en Los Ángeles era la completa antítesis de donde yo había estado el día anterior. Yo no podía creer lo caliente que estaba para un día de invierno. Esa mañana yo había tomado un vuelo sin retorno en avión a LA de Calgary, Canadá, el único hogar que yo había conocido durante mis once años de edad. Mientras el avión despegaba, mis ojos se llenaron de lágrimas. Yo no me quería mudar. Quería mucho a mi pueblo.

Después de que mi familia y yo llegamos a LAX, mis padres inmediatamente trataron de inscribirme en mi nuevo colegio. La junta del colegio nos informó que mi hermana y yo teníamos que hacernos los exámenes de tuberculosis. Mi papá caminó al Glendale Health Center a unas dos cuadras de mi nueva casa. Mientras esperábamos por nuestro turno, empecé a sentir la fatiga por la mudanza a un nuevo país esa mañana. Finalmente, llamaron mi número. Me senté enfrente de la enfermera, y mi mamá le entregó a ella mi record de inmunización de Canadá. La enfermera miró mi apellido y me empezó a realizar preguntas en un idioma que no era inglés. La miré a ella perpleja. Luego en inglés ella preguntó, "¿Eres Armenia verdad?" Yo moví mi cabeza de arriba abajo en señal de afirmación. Ella continuó, "¿No hablas el idioma?" Yo le dije que sí pero que no tenía idea de que ella estaba hablándome en el idioma armenio. Es' era un shock cultural. En Calgary, cuando la gente me pregur qué nacionalidad tenía, yo respondía Armenia. Usualmente se veían confundidos y decían, "¿Ah de Rumania?" Y en Calgary, cuando hablaba armenio con mi familia, era como nuestro propio secreto lenguaje que nadie más podía entender. Aquí en Glendale, la mayoría de los residentes de la ciudad así como el personal de enfermería en este Departamento de Salud eran armenios, pero yo no podía entender ni una sola palabra de lo que esta enfermera me estaba diciendo. La enfermera decidió hablar inglés. Luego, me enteré que esa enfermera me estaba hablando en otro dialecto armenio.

La enfermera luego miró a mi record de inmunización y dijo, "!Los canadienses no saben nada sobre inmunizaciones!" Esto realmente me ofendió. Yo había recibido la vacuna de la rubéola tan solo dos días antes en Calgary a fin de cumplir con todos los requisitos de mis vacunas. La enfermera sacó una serie de jeringas. Comenzó a prepararse para darme pinchazos en el brazo. Yo no entendí lo que ella me estaba haciendo. Le clavó a mi brazo una aguja, la vacuna del tétano. Ella me pinchó otra vez con otra vacuna. Finalmente, ella administró la inyección de TB. Todo pasó muy rápido. Me paré y caminé hacia donde estaba mi madre a fin de esperar por el turno de mi hermana. Mi hermana se sentó en la misma silla de tortura que yo me había sentado. De repente me sentí mareada. Yo abrí mi boca para explicárselo a mi madre, pero tan pronto lo hice mi cabeza comenzó a dar vueltas. Lo próximo que yo recuerdo fue despertarme, acostada en una mesa de examen con mis pies en el aire. El olor de sales de olores penetrantes irritó mi nariz. "¿Qué paso?" Resultó que tuve unas pequeñas convulsiones y me desmayé. Bienvenida a América. Por el siguiente par de días mi brazo estaba increíblemente adolorido por la vacuna del tétano. Yo casi no podía levantarlo. Después de que los exámenes de TB resultaron negativos fui autorizada a inscribirme en el colegio.

Rebobinando dieciséis años después cuando me tocaba ponerme otra vacuna del tétano, la evadí como a la plaga. Yo sabía que era importante recibirla pero mi experiencia pasada me dejó un sabor amargo en mi boca. No podía evadir la vacuna del tétano para siempre.

En el 2006, el Departamento de Salud del Condado de Miami-Dade estaba conduciendo su campaña de inmunización de empleados. Yo quería recibir la vacuna contra la gripe por lo que obtuve mi record de inmunización anterior de mi colegio de bachillerato. Yo esperé mientras colega tras colega recibía inmunizaciones y la vacuna contra la gripe. Luego fue mi turno. Me senté en la temida silla y entregué mi record de inmunizaciones. Estaba claro que yo debía haber recibido la vacuna del tétano mucho antes. Tenía los nervios destrozados. El miedo corría rampante a través de mi rígido cuerpo. Todo el personal de SIP (Proyecto de Inmunización Especial) estaba tratando de calmarme. Tracie, mi compañera de trabajo, trataba de distraerme mientras mi brazo era preparado para las vacunas. Para mi sorpresa, en un par de minutos todo había pasado. No me sentí mal. Además, mi brazo no estaba adolorido después.

La Primera Dama Eleonor Roosevelt lo dijo, "Tú adquieres fuerza, coraje y confidencia con cada experiencia en la que tú de verdad paras al ver miedo en la cara. Tu debes hacer lo que tu piensas que no puedes hacer." Esa cálida, húmeda tarde en Miami, se veía miedo en mi cara y adquirí seguridad en mi misma. ☀

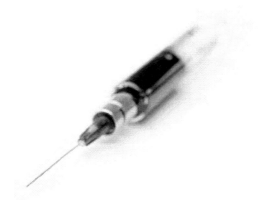

Yo te bali yon piki Laperèz

Por Amy Tejirian

Jou tyèd ak solèy nan mwa Fevrye nan Los Angeles la pa te menm bagay ditou ak kote mwen te ye jou lavèy la. Mwen pa te vle kwè ke li te kapab fè cho konsa yon jou ki te nan mwa fredi nan sezon ivè a. Jou maten sa a mwen te pran yon biye avyon pou ale sèlman lèke mwen te vwayaje pou Los Angeles paske mwen pa tap tounen nan Calvary nan Canada ki te kay mwen pandan onzan.

Lè mwen rive ak fanmi mwen nan aeropò Los Angeles, paran mwen te eseye anrejistre mwen menm moman an nan yon lekòl nan California. Gwoup moun ki reskonsab lekòl yo nan vil la, moun sa yo rele school board yo te di ke mwen ak sè mwen a te bezwen yon tès pou tibekilòz avan pou yo te aspete nou nan lekòl. Fanmi mwen ale nan sant sante Glendale la ki te nan kèk ri apre kay nèf kote nou te fèk vinn abite a. Pandan nou te ap tann tou pa nopu pou nou fè tès la mwen te santi fatig vwayaj mwen te fè nan peyi nèf la an maten sa a. Alafen yo rele nimewo mwen a. Mwen chita devan enfimyè a epi manman mwen lonje kat vaksen mwen a bali. Enfimyè a gade non mwen epi li komanse mande mwen keksyon nan yon lang ki pa te angle. Mwen gade li ak je mwen tankou je pwason fri. Epi lè sa a li mande mwen an angle «Ou se Armenyen pa vre ? »Mwen di li wi. Li kontinye ap pale lang la, mwen di li mwen pale Armenyen men mwen pa te gen okenn lide ke se te Armenyesn li te ap pale ak mwen. Se te yon sezisman pou mwen nan zafè lakilti paske nan Calvay lè yon moun te mande mwen moun ki peyi mwen te ye, mwen te konnen reponn yo Armeni epi yo te toujou parèt tankou moun ki pa te konpran sa mwen te di a epi yo te konnen di mwen «O ! Romanyen» Epi nan Calvary lè moun pale Armenyen ak fanmi mwen se te tankou yon lang sekrè ke okenn lòt moun pate kapab konprann. Isit la nan Glandale preske tout moun ki te abite la ak enfimyè nan depatman lasante a se te Armenyen men mwen pa te konprann yon sèl mo nan lang enfimyè sa a tap pale ak mwen. Enfimyè a te deside pou li pale angle, se apre sa ke mwen vinn konnen ke li te ap pale yon lòt lang Armenyen yo pale nan kèk pwovens nan peyi Armeni.

Enfimyè a te gade kat vaksen mwen a epi li di: «Kanadyen pa konnen anyen nan zafè vaksen » Sa pa te fè mwen plezi paske te gen 2 jou ke nan Calvary mwen te pran vaksen kont Ribeol pou ke mwen te kapab an règ ak tout vaksen mwen ki te nesesè. Enfimyè a rale yon bann zegwi, li te pa pare li pou li ban mwen yon vaksen nan bra. Mwen pa te konprann sa li te vle fè mwen a. Li pike mwen nan bra ak yon zegwi pou li ban mwen yon vaksen tetanòs, li pike mwen ankò ak yon lòt vaksen. Epi alafen li ban mwen piki pou tibekilòz la. Tout sa te pase twò vit. Mwen te kanpe epi mwen mache al jwen manman mwen pou mwen tann ke yo te fini ak sè mwen a. Sè mwen a te al chita nan menm chèz pou totire moun la kote mwen te fèk chita a. San atann mwen santi mwen toudi mwen te ap louvri bouch mwen pou mwen esplike manman mwen sa ki te ap pase mwen a men menm lè ke mwen te eseye louvri bouch mwen tèt mwen te tonbe vire. Dènye bagay ke mwen te sonje se ke mwen te ap eseye louvri je mwen alòske mwen te kouche sou yon tab konsiltasyon ak pye mwen anlè. Move zodè sèl amonyak te ap irite nen mwen. «Sa ki te pase ?» Li te rive ke mwen te gen yon ti kriz epi mwen te pèdi konesans. Bon vini nan Lèzetazini. Pou kèk jou an apre yo bra mwen te fè mwen mal akòz vaksen tetanòs la. Mwen pa te kapab leve li. Apre rezilta tès tibekilòz la te negatif yo te kite mwen ale lekòl.

Sèzan apre lè mwen te dwe pran yon lòt vaksen, mwen vinn sonje sa ki te pase a epi mwen te deside kabre zafè pran vaksen a.

Mwen te konnen ke vaksen se yon bagay enpòtan menm ak sa ki te pase 'm la te kite yon move souvni pou mwen. Mwen pa te kapab kontinye kabre vaksen tetanòs la pou tout tan.

An 2006, depatman sante piblik nan Miyami tap mache bay vaksen a la ronn badè. Mwen te vle pran vaksen pou grip flu a, kidonk mwen voye cheche kat vaksen mwen nan ansyen lekòl segondè mwen a. Mwen te tann apre tout lòt anplwaye nan travay la te finn pran vaksen yo ak vaksen grip la. Epi tou pa mwen te vinn rive. Mwen al chita nan chèz ke mwen te si tèlman pè a epi mwen lonje kanè vaksen mwen bay. Li te klè ke mwen te an reta anpil pou vaksen tetanòs mwen a. Mwen te te plen ak kè sote. Kò mwen te rèd ak laperèz. Tout moun ki travay nan pwogram vaksinasyon a yo rele SIP la tap eseye kalme mwen. Yon kanmarad nan travay la yo rele Tracie tap eseye fè mwen wete lide mwen sou zafè vaksen a pandan ke yo te ap netwaye bra mwen pou mwen pran vaksen a. Mwen te byen sezi pou mwen wè ke nan kèk minit tout bagay te fini. Mwen pa te menm konnen lè ke yo te pike mwen a. Epi apre bra mwen pa te fè mwen mal ditou.

Madanm yon prezidan Ameriken ki rele Eleanor Roosvelt te byen di sa ki pase mwen a nan pawòl sa yo:» Yon moun pran fòs ak kouraj epi li vini kwè nan tèt li lè ke li fè eksperyans kote li gade laperèz an fas. Yon moun dwe eseye fè tout bagay ke li kwè ke li pa kapab fè».

Nan apremidi chalè ak imidite nan Miyami a mwen te gade laperèz mwen a an fas epi mwen te vinn genyen konfyans nan tèt mwen.

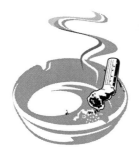

My Habit

By Mort Laitner

Getting Started...

As a 13 year-old growing up in the Catskill Mountains, I can remember smoking my first cigarette as if it were yesterday. Joel, Bobby, Donna, Rissa and I had concocted a plan to smoke our first cigarette. My friends and I thought it was cool to smoke. When do you get a chance to share hits with a pretty girl? We snuck into a rock formation called "Dead Man's Canyon" to smoke our parents' pilfered Newports, Marlboros, and Camels. The canyon consisted of two thirteen-foot-high by ten-foot-wide, thirty-thousand-pound boulders situated approximately eight feet apart. These boulders had been moved in place during the last great ice-age. Legend has it that either some Iroquois Indians carrying tomahawks and bows and arrows or a large brown bear was chasing a fur capped frontiersman who attempted to escape by leaping across the eight-foot gap. Slipping, he fell into the crevasse, hit his head, and broke his neck. Needless to say he died.

Dead Man's Canyon was the perfect place to hide and smoke a few cigarettes. Parents or police would hardly ever venture into this part of the wilderness. The first time we went there and every time after, we felt like adults as we inhaled the white menthol-flavored smoke. Even these filtered cigarettes caused us to cough as we felt the burning smoke enter our lungs.

Tobacco was our forbidden fruit. In those days my parents

smoked up to two packs a day. As a teenager, I distinctly remember my father, who was a medical doctor, waking up in the morning and going to the bathroom in his boxers to hack-up his lungs. The tobacco companies never offered my dad royalties for a TV commercial showing the phlegm dripping out of his mouth. You would think this memory alone would have taught me to not smoke. However, we were continually bombarded with advertisements of beautiful young models sitting next to flowing streams with the look of love in their eyes as they lit up. My other favorite was the ultra-macho Marlboro Cowboys riding stallions in red stone canyons and then resting with a Marlboro hanging off their lips. How could we simple teenagers not want to be these lucky people? And it was cheap. A pack cost as little as thirty-five cents; vices were so much cheaper in the good ole' days.

These were the days:
- A twelve year old could go into the corner grocery and buy a pack, no questions asked.
- Cigarettes were rarely called cancer sticks or nails in one's coffin.
- No one had even thought of the Great American Smokeout.
- The tobacco companies did not want us to know that smoking was the cause of approximately 80% of lung cancer deaths.
- The surgeon general was not warning us that, "Cigarette smoking may injure your health."
- Tobacco companies lied to us; never thinking they would get caught.
- Every media outlet made millions of dollars advertising cigarettes. Who could blame them for not telling the truth?
- Doctors in advertisements would recommend a particular brand of cigarettes.
- On a flight to Miami on Eastern Airlines, every passenger would get a cute-looking-mini- five-pack as a gratuity and of course for the industry to hook the unsuspecting with their poison. Hard to believe that people used to smoke on airplanes.
- Pregnant women were not warned of the dangers of smoking.

Getting hooked...

My habit through high school and college was limited to a few cigarettes a week. However by law school, with the pressure on, a half a pack-a-day was not unusual. By the time I was a lawyer with the Department of Health and Rehabilitative Services my office was filled with smoke to the point that my non-smoking secretary would cough every time she took dictation. Today, I feel guilty for my thoughtless behavior. I did not know the dangers of second-hand smoke.

By the early eighties, my boss, Dr. Richard Morgan, Director of the Miami-Dade County Health Department, was a key player in the Dade County Medical Association Anti-Tobacco drive. Doctors campaigned against smoking in the work place, smoking in health facilities, and the advertisement of tobacco products.

These were the days when:

My dad had an 8 inch Goodyear rubber tire ashtray on his medical office desk which almost always was stuffed with Camel butts.

Kick-Your-Habit nicotine chewing gum and sucking candy did not exist.

Many smokers collected Zippo lighters. My most treasured was the one with Joe Camel riding a motor cycle through New York City near the World Trade Center.

I also collected sterling-silver-cigarette cases and when I removed a cigarette from the shiny case I felt like a Hollywood silent film star in the nineteen twenties.

My next door neighbor, who was so addicted to the toxic weed, smoked even after he was diagnosed with emphysema. He would remove his oxygen mask light up even to the day he died.

Kicking the Habit....

One of the hardest things to do in my life was kicking my twenty year habit. One a.m. would find me in my closet with my hands in my sports-coat pockets scrounging for a cigarette to feed my habit.

I bummed cigarettes in the hopes of smoking less than a pack a day. My smoking friends now thought I was a pain in the butt. Quitting was made more difficult because my wife-- with a one cigarette a day habit-- always kept a pack in the house.

I tried the reward system in which for every day that I did not smoke, I would add a few dollars to the kitty to purchase a desired gift. However my daily one-hour drive home still required five cigarettes. Even with these gimmicks, I woke up coughing my lungs out-- just like my dad—at this moment, I knew I had to quit.

I can't remember my last cigarette, I know I sucked on nicorette candy and chewed nicorette gum for over two weeks. I knew that just like an alcoholic, I had to resolve that my lips, my tongue, my lungs would never again taste tobacco because if they did I would be hooked all over again.

I haven't smoked a cigarette in over 20 years.

As I now stand in Dead Man's Canyon remembering my boyhood, my parents, and my friends as I look at the chasm between the two large boulders, I realize when I smoked I was careening between the rocks. Luckily, I grabbed on to the ledge pulling myself onto the large stone when I kicked my deadly habit. However, my habit was not as lucky -- it died like the frontiersman.

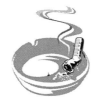

Mi Hábito

Por Mort Laitner

El Comienzo...

Como si hubiese sido ayer, puedo recordar fumando mi primer cigarrillo cuando tenía trece años y crecía en las Montañas de Catskill. Joel, Bobby, Donna, Rissa y yo habíamos concertado un plan para fumar nuestro primer cigarrillo. Mis amigos y yo pensamos que estaba muy en la onda fumar. ¿Cuándo tienes la oportunidad de compartir jalones con una muchacha bonita? Nos escondimos en una formación rocosa llamada "Dead Man's Canyon" a fin de fumar los hurtados Newports, Marlboros, y Camels de nuestros padres. El Cañón consistía en dos rocas grandes de treinta mil libras de trece pies de altura por diez pies de ancho, situadas aproximadamente a ocho pies de distancia. Estas grandes rocas habían sido movidas de lugar durante la última gran glaciación. La leyenda dice que bien algunos Indios Iroquois cargando un hacha de pelea, lazos y flechas, o bien un gran oso marrón, estaba persiguiendo un colonizador con una capucha de piel que intentaba escapar brincando a través de la abertura de ocho pies. Resbalándose, se cayó en la abertura, se pegó en la cabeza y se rompió el cuello. De más estar decir que él murió.

Dead Man's Canyon era el lugar perfecto para esconderse y fumar algunos cigarrillos. Los padres o la policía difícilmente se aventurarían hacia esta parte inhóspita. La primera vez que fuimos allí y las siguientes veces, nos sentimos como adultos mientras inhalábamos el humo blanco con sabor a mentol. Aun estos cigarrillos filtrados nos causaron toser cuando sentimos el ardiente humo entrar a nuestros pulmones.

El tabaco era nuestra fruta prohibida. Durante esos días mis padres se fumaban hasta dos paquetes al día. Como adolescente, yo claramente recuerdo a mi padre, quien era un doctor en medicina, parándose en la mañana y dirigiéndose al baño en sus calzoncillos a expectorar la flema de sus pulmones. Las compañías de tabaco nunca le ofrecieron a mi papá regalías por un comercial de televisión mostrando su flema saliendo de su boca. Tú podrías pensar que tan solo este recuerdo me hubiera enseñado a mí a no fumar. Sin embargo, fuimos continuamente bombardeados con anuncios publicitarios de modelos jóvenes bellas sentadas al lado del humo circulando con la mirada de amor en sus ojos mientras encendían un cigarrillo. Mi otro favorito eran los ultra-machos Vaqueros de Marlboro montando caballos sementales en las rocas rojas del cañón y luego descansando con un Marlboro puesto en sus labios. ¿Cómo no podríamos nosotros simples adolescentes querer ser una de estas personas con suerte? Y era barato. Un paquete costaba tan barato como treinta y cinco centavos; los vicios eran mucho más baratos en los buenos viejos tiempos.

Estos eran los días...
- Una persona de doce años podía ir a la tienda de la esquina, y comprar un paquete, sin hacérseles ninguna pregunta.
- Los cigarrillos fueron raramente llamados palitos de cáncer o clavos en el ataúd de uno.
- Nadie había pensado en el Día sin Tabaco en los Estados Unidos.
- Las compañías de tabaco no querían que nosotros supiéramos que fumar era la causa principal de aproximadamente 80% de las muertes de cáncer de pulmón.
- El Cirujano General no nos estaba advirtiendo que, "El fumar cigarrillos puede dañar tu salud."
- Las compañías de tabaco nos engañaron; nunca pensando que iban a ser agarradas.
- Cada medio de comunicación hizo millones de dólares haciendo anuncios de cigarrillos. ¿Quién puede culparlos por no haber dicho la verdad?
- Los doctores en anuncios recomendaban una marca particular de cigarrillos.
- En un vuelo a Miami en la línea aérea Eastern Airlines, cada pasajero recibía un bonito mini-paquete de cinco como un obsequio y por su puesto para la industria agarrar el

desprevenido con su veneno. Difícil pensar que las personas acostumbraban a fumar en los aviones.

• Las mujeres embarazadas no se les advertía de los peligros de fumar.

El caer en el vicio...

Mi hábito en bachillerato y la universidad estaba limitado a algunos cigarrillos por semana. Sin embargo en la escuela de leyes, con la presión encima, mitad de un paquete al día no era inusual. Para el momento de que era abogado con el Departamento de Salud y Servicios de Rehabilitación mi oficina estaba llena de humo hasta el punto que mi no fumadora secretaria tosía cada vez que recibía dictados. Hoy, me siento culpable por mi comportamiento desconsiderado. No sabía de los peligros del humo de segunda mano.

A principio de los ochentas, mi jefe, Dr. Richard Morgan, Director del Departamento de Salud del Condado de Miami-Dade, fue una pieza esencial en la campaña Anti-Tabaco de la Asociación Médica del Condado de Dade. Los doctores hicieron campaña en contra de fumar en el sitio de trabajo, en los establecimientos médicos, y de los anuncios de productos de tabaco.

Estos eran los días cuando:

Mi papá tenía un cenicero de rueda de goma de 8 pulgadas de Goodyear en el escritorio de su oficina médica el cual casi siempre estaba lleno de colillas de Camel.

Caramelos y gomas de mascar de nicotina para eliminar el hábito no existían.

Muchos fumadores coleccionaban encendedores de Zippo. Mi más preciado era el que tenía a Joe Camel conduciendo una motocicleta a través de la ciudad de Nueva York cerca del World Trade Center.

Yo también coleccionaba estuches de plata de esterlina y cuando yo sacaba un cigarrillo del brillante estuche me sentía como una estrella de película silenciosa de Hollywood en los mil novecientos veinte.

Mi vecino de al lado, quien estaba tan adicto a la tóxica hierba mala, fumó inclusive después de haber sido diagnosticado con enfisema. El se removía la máscara de oxígeno a fin de encender un cigarrillo inclusive hasta el día que murió.

Dejando el hábito...

Una de las cosas más difíciles que hice en mi vida fue dejar mi hábito de veinte años. Una a.m. me encontraba en mi closet con mis manos en los bolsillos de mis chaquetas deportivas gorroneando un cigarrillo para alimentar mi hábito.

Gorroneé cigarrillos con la esperanza de fumar menos de un paquete al día. Mis amigos fumadores pensaban que yo era un dolor en el trasero. Dejarlo era más difícil porque mi esposa – con un hábito de un cigarrillo al día – mantenía siempre un paquete en la casa.

Intenté el sistema de recompensa según el cual por cada día que no fumaba, yo añadía algunos dólares a mi alcancía para comprar un regalo deseado. Sin embargo mi diario manejo a casa de una hora todavía requería cinco cigarrillos. Aun con estas trampas, me levantaba expectorando toda la flema de mis pulmones –igual que mi papá- en ese momento. Yo sabía que debía dejarlo.

No puedo recordar mi último cigarrillo. Sé que chupé caramelos de nicotina y mastiqué goma de mascar de nicotina por más de dos semanas. Sabía que al igual que un alcohólico, debía resolver que mis labios, mi lengua y mis pulmones nunca más probarían el tabaco porque si lo hacían hubiese sido agarrado del todo nuevamente.

No he fumado un cigarrillo en más de veinte años.

Cuando ahora me paro en el Dead Man's Canyon recordando a mi niñez, a mis padres y a mis amigos, mientras miro el abismo entre las dos grandes piedras, me doy cuenta que mientras fumaba estaba brincando entre las rocas. Con suerte, me agarré del saliente empujándome a mi mismo sobre la grande roca cuando dejé mi mortal hábito. Sin embargo, mi hábito no tuvo la misma suerte – murió como el colonizador. ☀

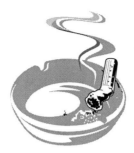

Move abitid mwen a

Lè ke mwen te komanse …

Kòm yon jenn moun trèzan ki te ap grandi nan Mòn Catskill yo, mwen sonje kòm si se te ayè lè mwen te fimen premye sigarèt mwen. Joel, Bobby, Donna, Rissa ak mwen nou te mete sou pye yon plan pou nou te fimen premye sigarèt nou.

Mwen menm ak zanmi mwen yo te te kwè ke se te yon bèl bagay lè yon moun fimen paske li te fè ou bròdè ak chèlbè. Ki lòt jan ou janm gen chans pou ou tande bèl mizik ak yon bèl ti fi? Nou foure kò nou nan yon twou wòch ki rele «Dead Man Canyon» (sa ki vle di falèz nan mitan mòn kote nonm la te mouri a) pou nou te fimen sigarèt Newport, Malboro, Camel ke nou te volè nan sigarèt fanmi nou.

Falèz nan mitan mòn la te fèt ak 2 gwo wòch ki te peze 30,000 liv epi te mezire 13 pye de wo ak dis pye nan lajè, falèz nan mitan 2 wòch yo te mezire yuit pye. Gwo wòch sa yo te deplase vinn chita kote yo ye a depi nan tan benmbo sa yo rele epòk latè a te jele ak glas «ice age». Lejand, kont ansyen yo rakonte ke te genyen gwoup endyen Irokwa ak hach yo ak flèch yo ki te monte sou de gwo lous mawon ki te ap kouri dèyè yon blan ki te kon achte po bèt sou fwontyè a. Blan sa a ki tap eseye chape poul li te vole pou li janbe yuit pye ki te separe 2 gwo wòch yo. Blan a te glise pye li te chape, li te tonbe nan falèz la li te frape tèt li epi li te kase kou li. Mwen pa bezwen pèdi tan mwen pou mwen di ou ke li te mouri.

Dead man Canyon, nan mòn ki te gen yon falèz nan mitan wòch yo se te pi bon kote pou nou te kache pou fimen kèk sigarèt. Pa te gen paran ni lapolis ki te ap vinn foure kò yo nan rakwen pèdi sa a.

Premye fwa nou te ale la epi chak fwa an apre sa nou te santi nou te gran moun chak fwa ke nou te rale lafimen ki te gen gou mant la. Menm si sigarèt yo te gen filt ladan yo nou te touse kan menm lè nou te santi lafimen cho a antre nan poumon nou. Yo te defann nou fimen tabak tankou yo te di adan ak èv pa manje pòm la. Nan epòk sa a paran mwen yo te fimen jiska 2 pòch sigarèt pa jou. Kòm jenn moun ki pa te gen ventan mwen byen sonje papa mwen ki se te yon doktè ki te leve chak maten ap touse nan sal de ben a pou li netwaye poumon li.

Konpanyi tabak la pa janm ofri papa mwen lajan pou li te fè reklam nan televizyon kote yo ap montre flèm ki ap koule sot nan bouch li. Ou ta kwè ke souvni bagay sa sèlman tap kont pou montre mwen ke pou mwen pa fimen paske li pa bon pou la sante. Tout okontrè yo te bonbade nou ak foto bèl rivyè ki te ap koule kote bèl manken te chita ak lanmou nan je yo lè ke yo ap limen yon sigarèt. Reklam ke mwen te renmen pase tout lòt yo se te kòbòy Malboro a ki te tèlman matcho lè li te monte chwal li nan laplenn nan mitan mòn yo epi ki te al repoze li apre kous chwal la ak yon sigarèt Malboro pandye nan bouch li.

Kijan ou ta vle ke nou menm jenn moun pa te reve pou nou sanble ak moun sa yo ki te gen bèl chans sa yo? Epi sigarèt yo te bon mache. Yon pòch sigarèt te koute yon ti kras kòb tankou 35 santim. Vis sigarèt la te tèlman pi bon mache nan bon vye tan lontan.

Men sa ki te konn pase nan bon vye tan lontan:
- yon ti moun douzan te kapab al nan boutik nan kwen a epi li achte yon pòch sigarèt san yo pa mande li okenn keksyon.
- Yo preske pa te janm rele sigarèt ti bagèt ki bay kansè oswa klou nan sèkèy moun.
- Pa te genyen yon moun ki te janm sonje pou li fè yon jou kote li tap mande tout ameriken pou pou yo pa fimen ditou.
- Konpanyi ki vann tabak yo pa te vle nou konnen ke fimen sigarèt te lakòz ke sou chak 100 moun ki te mouri ak kansè nan poumon 80 ladan yo te mouri paske yo te fimen sigarèt.
- Moun ki reskonsab lasante ak edikasyon moun sou zafè lasante ke yo rele surgeon general nan peyi ameriken pa te janm avèti nou sou koze sa a. Yo pa te janm di nou ke fimen sigarèt te kapab fè moun malad.

- Konpanyi ki vann tabak yo te ba nou manti, paske yo pa te konprann ke yo te ap finn pa kenbe yo yon jou.
- Tout konpanyi ki fè reklam yo te ranmase milyon dola nan fè reklam pou sigarèt. Eske ou te kapab ba yo tò deske yo pa te di nou laverite a ?
- Doktè ki te ap pale nan reklam yo lè sa a te menm di moun ke te genyen yon mak sigarèt ki te bon pou moun fimen.
- Le pasaje yo te monte avyon Eastern Airlines yo ki te pral nan miyami yo te konn ba yo gratis yon ti pake sigarèt ki te genyen senk sigarèt ladan yo epi tankou nou konprann li se te yon jan pou yo te fè moun sa yo ki pa te remake anyen komanse fimen pwazon yo rele sigarèt la. yon vis ke yo pa tap ka kite fasilman. Li menm difisil pou moun kounye a kwè ke moun te konn fimen nan avyon.
- Yo pa te janm di fanm ansent ke te genyen danje pou lasante yo ak lasante ti bebe yo si fanm la fimen lè li ansent.

Ki jan mwen pran vis la...

Lè mwen te nan lekòl segondè ak lè mwen te komanse nan inivèsite mwen te konn fimen sèlman kèk sigarèt nan yon semenn. Men lè ke mwen te komanse etidye nan lekòl de dwa pou mwen vini yon avoka, ak presyon lekòl la te mete sou mwen, mwen te konn fimen mwatye yon pòch sigarèt pa jou. Lè ke mwen te rive yon avoka ki te ap travay ak depatman lasante ak sèvis reabilitasyon biwo mwen a te tèlman plen ak lafimen ke sekretè ki te ap pran nòt ke mwen te ap dikte pou yo tape yo te ap touse chak fwa yo te ap travay bokote mwen. Kounye a mwen santi mwen koupab pou jan ke mwen te konpòte mwen ak yo. Mwen pa te konnen danje ki te genyen lè yon moun ap respire lafimen sigarèt ke lòt moun ap fimen.

Nan lane katreven yon patron mwen doktè Richard Morgan ki te direktè depatman lasante nan Miyami a se te yon manb ki te aktif anpil nan asosiyasyon doktè nan Ded Konti ki t ap lite pou moun pa sèvi ak tabak. Doktè yo te ap fè kanpay pou moun pa fimen nan kote yo ap travay, nan kote yo ap bay sèvis lasante, epi tou pou konpanyi tabak yo sispan fè reklam pou tabak.

Se te epòk lè ke:

Papa mwen te genyen yon sandriye yuit pous ki te anfòm yon

kaoutchou Good Year ki te toujou plen ak pòy sigarèt Camel sou biwo li nan klinik li a.

Lè sa a chiklèt ki ak nikotin tabak ladan yo pou ede moun kite abitid fimen a epi tou manje sirèt pou ou pa fimen pa te existe.

Anpil moun ki te fimen te fè koleksyon brikè zippo. Sa mwen te pi renmen a se te yon ki te genyen Joe Camel ki te ap monte yon motosiklèt nan Nou Yòk bokote World Trade Center a.

Mwen te fè koleksyon bwat sigarèt ki fèt an ajan epi lè ke mwen te pran yon sigarèt pou mwen fimen nan bwat klere sa a mwen te santi mwen te tankou yon aktè nan film sinema bèbè yo ki te konn pase nan epòk 1920 a.

Vwazen a kote mwen a ki pa te kapab viv li menm tou san zèb pwazon a, te kontinye fimen menm apre ke li te fè maladi anfizèm nan poumon li. Li te konn retire mask oxijèn la pou li limen sigarèt la jouk jou ke li te mouri a.

Kite move abitid...

Yon nan bagay ki te pi di pou mwen fè nan vi mwen se te kite move abitid mwen te genyen pandan ventan. A inè di maten map chèche yon sigarèt nan pòch espòt jakèt mwen pou mwen kontinye ak move abitid mwen a.

Mwen pa te gen kè kontan akòz de move eksperyans mwen ak sigarèt la, mwen te fache ak sigarèt la paske konsa mwen te espere ke mwen ta va fimen mwens ke yon pòch sigarèt pa jou. Zanmi mwen yo ki te gen abitid fimen yo te pran mwen pou yon enmèdan lè sa a. Li te pi difisil pou mwen kite fimen akòz de madanm mwen ki se te yon moun ki te abitye fimen yon grenn sigarèt chak jou, epi ki te toujou gen yon pòch sigarèt nan kay la. Mwen te eseye sistèm rekonpans la kote pou chak jou ke mwen pa te fimen mwen te mete kèk dola nan bwat sekrè mwen pou mwen achte yon kado ke mwen te vle genyen anpil.

Men pou mwen te kondwi pandan inè de tan pou al nan travay mwen chak jou mwen te bezwenn senk sigarèt. Menm lè ke mwen te eseye tout mannigèt sa yo mwen te leve an maten ap touse poumon mwen yo. Menm jan ak papa mwen, mwen te konnen lè sa a ke fòk mwen te kite fimen. Mwen pa sonje kilè mwen fimen dènye sigarèt mwen a Mwen konnen ke mwen te souse sirèt Nicorette pou fè moun kite fimen epi ke mwen te moulen chiklèt Nicorette pou plis ke de semenn. Mwen te konnen ke menm jan ak yon tafyatè fòk mwen te pran rezolisyon pou bouch mwen, lang mwen ak poumon mwen pa janm touche ak gou tabak la ankò sinon mwen ta va rekònmanse tounen esklav fimen sigarèt la ankò.

Mwen pa janm fimen yon sigarèt ankò depi ventan.

Kounye a ke mwen kanpe nan Dead Man Canyon a, falèz nan mitan mòn kote nonm la te mouri a, epi ke map sonje lè mwen te jenn, ke map sonje paran mwen ak zanmi mwen yo, lè mwen ap gade gwosè falèz ki nan mitan de gwo ròch yo mwen realize ke lè mwen te ap fimen a mwen tap pandye sou falèz la. Erèzman mwen te rale kò mwen monte sou sou ròch la, lè ke mwen te sispan move abitid ki tap mennen mwen nan chemen lanmò. Men move abitid mwen a pate gen chans paske li menm tou li mouri tankou blan ki te konn achte po bèt sou fwontyè a. ☼

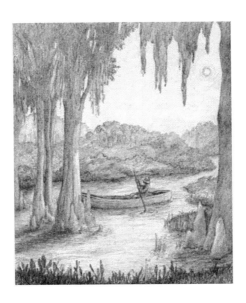

On The Wings of Angels

By Paula Mooty
Original Artwork by Vicki F. MootyJones

As I sat in the cemetery on a cool October evening, inhaling the sweet fragrance of jasmine, my eyes squinted as the golden evening sun touched the outstretched wings of cemetery angels. Suddenly, I spied two familiar names on a tombstone. The names were Victoria and Thomas Taylor. This reminded me of a story told by my Grandmother, Eliza Downing.

Around the late 1800's, the Taylors and the Downings started families in the small town of Fernandina which lies across the river from Jacksonville. At that time, Florida was only a state of sand, sea, and swamps. One weekend in June 1888, the Taylors and Downings gathered to discuss the qualities of summers in Florida: the heat, humidity, rain, disease and the inevitable hurricanes. They spoke about yellow fever, malaria, cholera, smallpox, dengue fever and consumption (tuberculosis). The ominous conversations were sweetened with fresh, coollemonade but the sour taste of fear lay heavy as they rested their heads on their pillows that night. In the depth of the evening, my great aunt Maggie Downing, a young teen, awoke with a fever, sweats, nausea and a headache. She wondered if she had food poisoning. By morning, she was dehydrated and weak from lack of sleep. Her parents rushed her to the family doctor. Maggie had been sick before but never like this.

After hitching up the carriage, crossing the river by ferry, and traveling for two hours, the family reached Jacksonville. They hurried to Dr. Brown's office. Dr. Brown diagnosed yellow fever. They knew the effect this news would have on Maggie, not to mention the community. Under a blanket of secrecy, Dr. Brown transferred Maggie to Jacksonville's St. Luke's Hospital.

As Maggie's temperature rose, her skin turned a yellow-green color. Maggie experienced intestinal bleeding and vomiting. In her delirium, she hallucinated eating with her brothers and sister on the veranda of their big house. Maggie's siblings were breakfasting on fresh blueberries, milk, and buttered biscuits covered with homemade strawberry jam. She imagined that she was going to the wharf to watch the schooners set sail. She envisioned the cool sea breezes and tasted the salty air while beads of sweat ran down her face. In her hospital bed, Maggie lay fighting the Angel of Death.

She won. Maggie was fortunate; she was well enough to go home after a month in the hospital. Before her release, four more cases were secretly admitted to St. Luke's. This was the beginning of the epidemic. Jacksonville business leaders feared if the epidemic news leaked, the city would go bankrupt. They decided this news had to be kept from the public. They would have to contain this disease. Dr. Brown contacted Dr. Andrew Downing, Maggie's brother, to be his assistant. As Andrew learned of the details of the disease, he knew that he must be part of the solution to help those in the same predicament as his sister.

Dr. Joseph Yates Porter, a medical officer with the U.S. Marine Hospital Service, was contacted to help curtail the outbreak. He was known for his work with the yellow fever epidemics in Key West. Dr. Porter had success in arresting the spread of the disease the previous year because his experience had led him to believe that the sick needed to be isolated from one another. Dr. Porter noticed that recovered patients were able to work with ill patients without being reinfected. He applied this strategy in fighting this grave disease.

If quarantine were to be declared in Jacksonville, there would be no safe haven for those fleeing the city to take refuge. Doctors Downing, Brown and Porter contacted the U.S. Public Health Service and the Red Cross for aid. Relief came in the guise of $200,000 from the U.S. Government and arrival of the Red Cross. Dr. Porter requested that a registered nurse, Jane Delano, be summoned to assist during the epidemic. She worked in the hospital organizing treatment of patients.

Dr. Downing flipped through ten years of ledger of Fernandina residences. He glanced at his silver pocket watch and noticed he had been searching for three hours. He found thirty-five survivors of the 1877 epidemic. Would they be willing to help care for the current yellow fever victims? Twenty-five survivors accepted the call of duty. Late in the afternoon, the brave twenty-five gathered outside Fernandina's public school for their departure. After a blessing by the Methodist minister, they set out for Jacksonville on horseback, ox cart and carriage.

The Jacksonville inhabitants panicked when the news of Yellow Fever "leaked." Even though the city's 26,000 citizens were already under quarantine, a mass exodus commenced. People fled in the dark of night on foot, horseback, steamer, train, boat, carriage, or ox cart to get away from the "Yellow Jack." Deputies on horseback carrying yellow flags (the quarantine flag) and sharp-shooter rifles were positioned to prevent the populace from entering or leaving without a special pass. Gunfire echoed as refugees crossed the temporary boundaries.

The city was under marshal law from dusk to dawn; a curfew was signaled by the loud boom of a cannon. Food became scarce, stores and hotels closed; social events and mail ceased. Mail was fumigated and lime was spread on the streets in an effort to contain the disease's spread. Bonfire flames lit the evening sky fueled by clothing and bedding.

Many residents escaped, some were shot and others turned back when confronted. Thousands became sick and hundreds died. When would this nightmare end? Jacksonville was a city under siege.

As the chill of the November morning settled on the Downing house, Maggie, home for a few months and still weak from her bout with Yellow Jack, finished setting the table when Papa Downing and Doc Andrew walked through the front door. Wearily, they entered the dining room and with a great sigh of relief made the long anticipated announcement, "No new cases have been reported for more than ten days. It looks like the epidemic is over."

Mother and Hattie, the housekeeper, ran into the room when they heard the news. Mother cried and hugged Papa. As they sat around the table, they thanked God for the deliverance from the yellow fever epidemic. The epidemic of 1888 finally came to an end after the first winter freeze having eliminated the mosquito population. The final count was 5,000 cases and 500 dead.[1]

As darkness blanketed the cemetery, I pictured an angel carrying brave men like Doc Reed and Doc Porter on its outstretched wings. I realized that public health servants are doing the work of angels on earth.

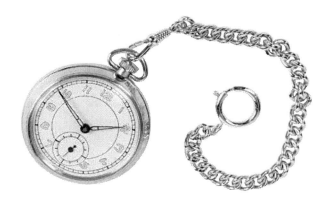

<hr />

1 On August 27, 1900, an Army physician, James Carroll, allowed an infected mosquito to feed on him. He developed a severe case of yellow fever which allowed his colleague, Dr. Walter Reed, to prove the dreaded disease was transmitted by mosquitoes. Yellow fever was the first human virus to be isolated and classified as a virus. Dr. Porter became Florida's first State Health Officer in 1888. The State Board of Health of Florida was established in 1889. The vector of yellow fever, Aedes aegypti, was discovered in 1900 by U.S. Army physicians. In 1927, the causative agent of yellow fever, Flaviavirus, was isolated and identified by Dr. Walter Reed. This discovery led to the development of a vaccine in 1937. Jane Delano, R.N., a distant relative of Franklin Delano Roosevelt, was a volunteer for the Army Reserve Corps ("ARC") and established the Nursing Corp for the American Red Cross in 1909-1912; The Nursing Corp enabled the United States to enter the First World War with a ready team of nurses numbering eight-thousand.

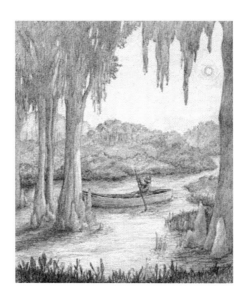

Sobre las alas de los angeles

Por Paula Mooty
Original de Trabajo Artístico por Vicki F. Mooty-Jones

Mientras estaba sentada en el cementerio en una tarde fría de Octubre, inhalando las dulces fragancias de jazmín, mis ojos echaban un vistazo mientras el dorado sol del atardecer tocaba las extendidas alas de los ángeles del cementerio. De repente, divisé dos nombres familiares en una lápida. Los nombres eran Victoria y Thomas Taylor. Esto me recordó a mí de una historia que me contó my Abuela, Eliza Downing.

Alrededor de finales de los 1800s, los Taylors y los Downings comenzaron familias en el pueblo pequeño de Fernandina, el cual queda al pasar el río de Jacksonville. En ese tiempo, Florida era solo un Estado de arena, mar y pantanos. Un fin de semana en Junio de 1888, los Taylors y los Downings se reunieron a discutir la calidad de los veranos en la Florida: el calor, la humedad, la lluvia, enfermedades y los inevitables huracanes. Ellos hablaron sobre la fiebre amarilla, malaria, cólera, viruela, fiebre de dengue y tuberculosis. La conversación de mal presagio estaba endulzada con limonada fría fresca pero el agrio sabor del miedo pesaba mientras ellos descansaban sus cabezas sobre las almohadas esa noche. Adentrada la noche, mi tía abuela Maggie Downing, una joven adolescente, se despertó con fiebre, sudor, nausea y dolor de cabeza. Se preguntó si tendría una intoxicación alimenticia. En la mañana, ella estaba deshidratada y débil por falta de sueño. Los padres la llevaron corriendo al médico de cabecera. Maggie había estado enferma antes pero nunca así.

Después de enganchar el carro al caballo, cruzar el río por ferry, y viajar por dos horas, la familia llegó a Jacksonville. Fueron rápidamente a la oficina del Dr. Brown. El Dr. Brown diagnosticó fiebre amarilla. Ellos sabían los efectos que la noticia sobre Maggie y la comunidad. Bajo una manta secreta, el Dr. Brown transfirió a Maggie al St. Luke's Hospital de Jacksonville.

Mientras la temperatura de Maggie subía, su piel adquirió un color verde-amarillento. Maggie experimentó sangramiento intestinal y vómito. En su delirio, ella alucinó estar comiendo con sus hermanos y hermanas en la galería de su gran casa. Los hermanos de Maggie estaban desayunando arándanos, leche y panecillos enmantequillados cubiertos con mermelada de fresa hecha en casa. Ella imaginó ir al muelle a ver los barcos de vela partir. Se imaginó los vientos fríos del mar y degustó el salado aire mientras gotas de sudor se deslizaban por su cara. En su cama de hospital, Maggie estaba combatiendo el Ángel de la Muerte.

Ella ganó. Maggie fue afortunada; ella estaba lo suficientemente bien para irse a casa después de un mes en el hospital. Antes de su salida del hospital, cuatro otros casos fueron secretamente admitidos al St. Luke Hospital. Este era el comienzo de la epidemia. Los líderes de negocio de Jacksonville temían que si la noticia de la epidemia se regaba, la ciudad se iría en bancarrota. Ellos decidieron que esta noticia debía ser mantenida fuera del público. Ellos tendrían que contener esta enfermedad. El Dr. Brown contactó al Dr. Andrew Downing, el hermano de Maggie, a fin de que fuera su asistente. Mientras el Dr. Andrew se informaba de los detalles de la enfermedad, él sabía que él debía formar parte de la solución a fin de ayudar a los que estaban en la misma situación de su hermana.

El Dr. Joseph Yates Porter, un oficial médico del Servicio de

Hospital de la Marina de los Estados Unidos, fue contactado para ayudar a reducir el brote. El era conocido por su trabajo contra la epidemia de fiebre amarilla en Key West. Dr. Porter tuvo éxito en contener la propagación de la enfermedad de años anteriores porque su experiencia lo llevó a creer que el enfermo debía ser aislado de los demás. El Dr. Porter notó que los pacientes que se habían recuperado eran capaces de trabajar con pacientes enfermos sin ser reinfectados. El aplicó esta estrategia al luchar contra esta grave enfermedad.

Si la cuarentena debía ser declarada en Jacksonville, no iba a haber lugar seguro para aquellos que escaparan la ciudad para obtener refugio. Los doctores Downing, Brown y Porter contactaron al Servicio de Salud Pública de los Estados Unidos y a la Cruz Roja para ayuda. El auxilio vino en la forma de $200,000.00 del gobierno de los Estados Unidos y el arribo de la Cruz Roja. Dr. Porter pidió que una enfermera registrada, Jane Delano, fuera convocada a asistir durante la epidemia. Ella trabajaba en el hospital organizando el tratamiento de los pacientes.

El Doctor Downing chequeó diez años de los archivos de los residentes de Fernandina. Echó un vistazo a su reloj de bolsillo plateado, y notó que el había estado buscando por tres horas. Encontró treinticinco sobrevivientes de la epidemia de 1877. ¿Estarían ellos dispuestos a ayudar a las actuales víctimas de fiebre amarilla? Veinticinco sobrevivientes respondieron a la llamada de servicio. Avanzada la tarde, los valientes veinticinco se reunieron a fuera del colegio público de Fernandina para su partida. Después de recibir la bendición del ministro metodista, salieron hacia Jacksonville a caballo, carretas de bueyes y carruajes.

Los habitantes de Jacksonville se llenaron de pánico cuando las noticias sobre la Fiebre Amarilla se esparcieron. Aun y cuando los 26,000 residentes de la ciudad estaba ya bajo cuarentena, un éxodo masivo comenzó. La gente huyó durante la oscuridad de la noche a pie, a caballo, en barco de vapor, tren, bote, carruaje, o carros de bueyes a fin de alejarse del "Yellow Jack". Los ayudantes del Sheriff a caballo cargaban banderas amarillas (la bandera de la cuarentena) y rifles de alta precisión fueron posicionados a fin de prevenir que la población entrara o saliera sin un pase especial. Los disparos hicieron eco mientras los refugiados cruzaron los límites temporales.

La ciudad estaba bajo la ley marcial desde el amanecer al anochecer; un toque de queda estaba señalizado por el estruendo de un cañón. La comida escaseaba; las tiendas y los hoteles cerraron; los eventos sociales y el correo cesaron. El correo fue fumigado y lima fue regado sobre las calles a fin de contener la propagación de la enfermedad. Llamas de hogueras iluminaron el cielo del anochecer cuyo combustible era la ropa de vestir y ropa de cama.

Muchos residentes escaparon, algunos fueron heridos de bala y otros se regresaron cuando fueron confrontados. Miles se enfermaron y cientos murieron. ¿Cuándo terminaría este infierno? Jacksonville era una ciudad sitiada.

Mientras el frío de la mañana de noviembre se asentó sobre la casa de los Downing, Maggie, de vuelta a casa por varios meses y todavía débil por su combate con Yellow Jack, terminó de poner la mesa cuando el Papa Downing y el Doctor Andrew caminaron a través de la puerta de enfrente. Con cansancio, entraron al comedor y con un gran suspiro de alivio hicieron el gran anticipado anuncio, "Por más de diez días, no se han reportado nuevos casos. Parece que la epidemia ha terminado."

La Madre y Hattie, la ama de llaves, corrieron hacia el comedor cuando oyeron la noticia. La Madre lloró y abrazó a Papá. Mientras se sentaban alrededor de la mesa, ellos dieron gracias a Dios por haberlos librado de la epidemia de fiebre amarilla. La epidemia de 1888 finalmente terminó después de la primera helada que erradicó la población de mosquito. El conteo final dio 5,000 casos y 500 muertes.[1]

Mientras la oscuridad cobijaba al cementerio, me imaginé a un ángel cargando valientes hombres como al Doctor Reed y Doctor Porter en sus abiertas alas. Me di cuenta que los trabajadores de salud pública están haciendo el trabajo de ángeles en la tierra.

---

1 El 27 de agosto de 1900, un médico de la Armada, James Carrol, permitió que un mosquito infectado lo picara. Desarrolló un caso severo de fiebre amarilla lo cual permitió a su colega, Dr. Walter Reed, probar que la temida enfermedad era transmitida por mosquitos. La fiebre amarilla fue el primer virus humano que fue aislado y clasificado como virus. El Dr. Porter se convirtió en el primer Oficial de Salud Pública en 1888. La Junta Estadal de Salud de la Florida fue establecida en 1889. El vector de fiebre amarilla, Aedes aegypti, fue descubierto en 1900 por médicos de la Armada. En 1927, el agente causante de fiebre amarilla, Flavivirus, fue aislado e identificado por el Dr. Waler Reed. Este descubrimiento condujo al desarrollo de la vacuna en 1937. Jane Delano, R.N., una familiar distante de Franklin Delano Roosevelt, fue una voluntaria del Army Reserve Corps ("ARC") y estableció el Nursing Corp de la Cruz Roja Americana en 1909-1912. El Nursing Corp permitió a los Estados Unidos entrar a la Primera Guerra Mundial con un equipo listo de ocho mil enfermeros.

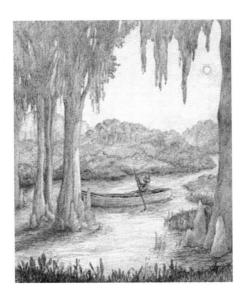

Sou Zèl Zanj Yo

Se Paula Mooty Ki ekri istwa sa a.
Se Vicki F. Mooty Jones ki pentire tablo sa a pou istwa a.

Pandan ke mwen te chita nan simityè a nan yon jou apremidi mwa oktòb ki te fè fre. Mwen te ap respire pafen jasmen ki te syav, je mwen te ap pich pich lè solèy koulè lò a nan apremidi sa a te poze sou zèl tou louvri zanj nan simityè a. Brid sou kou san atann mwen apèsi sou ròch ki make tomb la de non moun ke mwen te konnen. Non sa yo se te Victoria ak Thomas Taylor. Sa te fè mwen sonje yon istwa ke grann mwen Eliza Downing te rakonte mwen.

Nan fen lane 1800 yo moun Taylor yo ak moun Downing yo te kòmanse ap derape lafanmi yo nan ti vil ki rele Fernandina ki chita sou larivyè Jacksonville la.

Lè sa a Florida se te yon eta ki te fèt ak sèlman sab ak lanmè epi marekaj. Yon fen semen nan mwa Jen 1888, lafanmi Taylor ak Downing yo te rasanble pou yo diskite sou kijan epòk chalè nan mwa vakans yo te ye nan Florida: chalè, imidite, lapli, maladi epi siklòn yo ki pa te janm manke. Yo pale de lafièv jon, de malarya, de kolera, de maladi vèrèt, lafièv deng, epi sa yo rele konsompsyon sa ki te vle di tibekilòz. Kalite konvèsasyon sa yo ki te tout kote nan bouch tout moun te sikre ak bon jan limonad fre ki te fèk fèt men gou anmè laperèz la te peze lou lè ke yo te mete tèt yo sou zòrye pou yo te al domi jou swa sa a. Pandan ke li te finn nannwit nèt gran matant mwen Maggie Downing ki se te yon jenn moun lè sa a te leve ak yon lafyèv, li tap sye, li te gen kè plen epi li te gen maltèt. Li tap mande tèt li si li te manje yon manje gate ki te mete movè pwodwi nan kò li. Lè li leve an maten kò li te pèdi dlo li epi li te fèb paske li te pase nwit la san domi. Paran li yo te kouri mennen li lakay doktè lafanmi a. Maggie te konn malad avan sa men li pa te janm byen mal konsa.

Apre yo sele bèt yo nan bogi a, yo janbe larivyè a nan bato epi vwayaje pandan dezèdetan , fanmi a te rive Jacksonville. Yo te kouri nan klinik doktè Brown. Doktè Brown te di ke se te lafyèv jòn. Yo te konnen efè nouvel sa a ta pral genyen sou Maggie san konte sou moun nan kominote a . Avèk anpil sekrè doktè Brown fè entène Maggie nan lopital St Lukes nan Jacksonville.

Kòm tanperati Maggie tap monte, koulè po li te vini jòn tire sou vèt Maggie te ap senyen andedan vant li epi li te ap vomi. Pandan ke li te ap delire li fè vizyon ke li te ap manje ak frè ak sè li yo sou veranda nan gwo kay yo a. Frè ak sè Maggie yo te ap manje manje maten yo ki se te mi ki te fèk keyi, lèt, biskwit ki te fèt ak bè epi ki te kouvri ak konfiti frèz ke yo te fè lakay la. Maggie te ap imajine tèt li ki te pral sou waf la pou gade bato avwal yo ki tap pran vwal. Li te ap fè vizyon yon briz lanmè fre epi li te ap imajine ke li tap goute sèl ki te nan lè a alòse se te gout syè ki tap kouri sou figi li nan lopital la.. Men se te nan kaban lopital li a ke Maggie te kouche ap lite kont zanj lanmò a.

Maggie te pote laviktwa sou maladi ak lanmò, li te genyen anpil chans ke li te refè ase pou li te ka retounen lakay li apre ke li te pase yon mwa nan lopital la. Avan yo te exeate li te genyen kat lòt ka lafièv jòn yo te fè antre an sekrè nan lopital la. Se te komansman yon epidemi . Moun ki te reskonsab biznis yo nan vil Jacksonville te gen laperèz ke si nouvèl epidemi a te pran lari vil la te ap tonbe anfayit . Yo deside ke piblik la pa te pou konnen di tou nouvèl ke te gen epidemi a. Yo te dwe fè jefò pou anpeche maladi a gaye.

Doktè Brown te kontakte doktè Andrew Downing ki se frè Maggie pou li vinn asistan li nan lit kont epidemi a. Lè ke doktè Andrew finn konnen tou detay sou zafè maladi a li te konnen ke li te oblije ede jwen yon solisyon pou ede moun ki te nan menm sitiyasyon ke sè li

Maggie te ye avan li te geri a.. Yo kontakte doktè Joseph Yates Porter, ki te yon doktè nan lame nan sèvis lopital marin ameriken, pou li ede anpeche maladi a gaye. Yo te byen konnen bon jan kalite travay doktè sa a te fè ak epidemi lafyèv jòn nan Key West. Doktè Porter te gen anpil siksè nan anpeche maladfi a gaye nan ane ki te fèk pase a paske eksperyans li te fè li kwè ke moun malad yo te dwe nan izolasyon pou yo pa te malanje ak lòt moun pandan yo malad la. Doktè Porter te wè tou ke moun ki te malad yo epi ki te refè anba maladi a te kapab travay ak moun malad yo san ke yo pa tonbe malad ankò. Se plan sa a ke doktè Porter te pral mete sou pye pou lite kont maladi grav sila a.

Si yo te deklare karantèn pou moun pa antre ak soti nan vil la, Jacksonville pa tap genyen yon kote ansekirite pou akeyi moun moun ki tap kouri sove kite zòn la. Doktè downing Brown ak Porter te mande Lakwarouj ak sèvis sante piblik ameriken ede yo ak epidemi a. Gouvènman te voye 200,000 dola pou ede yo epi travayè Lakwarouj te presante yo tou. Doktè Porter mande pou enfimyè Jane Delano ki gen diplòm li anregistre ak leta vinn ede ak epidemi a. Li te pral travay nan lopital la pou òganize tretman patyan yo.

Doktè Downing feyte dis paj rejis kay tout fanmi ki te nan Fernandina yo. Li gade mont an ajan moun lontan te konn mete nan pòch yo ke li te genyen epi li wè ke li te pase twazè ap cheche. Li jwenn trantsenk moun ki te pase maladi a nan epidemi 1877 la epi ki pa te mouri. Eske yo te ap vle ede pran swen moun ki te malad ak lafyèv jòn kounye a? Tout transenk moun ki te chape anba lanmò ak lafyèv jòn la te asepte ede lè ke yo te mande yo èd yo. Nan apremidi a lè ke li te preske nannwit trantsenk moun brav yo te rasanble devan lekòl piblik Fernandina a pou yo te ale fè vwayaj la. Apre ke pastè metodist la te beni yo, yo te derape pou ale Jacksonville sou chwal, charèt bèf ap tire, ak bogi. Moun nan vil Jacksonville te pran laperèz lè yo wè ke nouvèl epidemi lafyèv jòn la te pran lari. Menm lè ke 26,000 sitwayen vil la te deja sou karantèn, yon ekzòd te kòmanse, yon pil moun te ap kouri kite vil la. Moun te ap sove nan mitan lannwit la kèk a pye kèk sou chwal, sou bato ki mache ak vapè dlo, tren, bato, bogi, charèt bèf, pou yo te ale lwen lafyèv jòn la ke yo te rele «Yellow Jack » Militè ki te monte sou chwal ki te kenbe drapo jòn ki lè sa a te drapo pou mete yon kote nan karantèn, te gen fizi yo nan men yo tou, militè yo te mete yo nan pozisyon pou pou yo tire pou anpeche popilas la antre oswa soti si yo pa te genyen yon pèmisyon espesyal nan men yo. Kout zam tap sonnen lè refijye yo tap travèse baryè pwovizwa ke militè yo te trase otou vil la.

Vil la te anba lwa masyal depi solèy kouche jouktan li leve, yo te anonse kouvrefe a ak gwo bwi yon kout kanon. Manje te vini ra magazen ak lotèl yo te fèmen. Lapost te sispan fonksyonen epi tout aktivite sosyal te sispan tou. Yo te espre lèt moun ekri ak resewa ak pwodwi dezenfektan epi yo te simen sitwon nan tout lari pou yo te fe yon jèfò pou anpeche maladi a gaye. Flanm dife bagay yo te ap boule tankou rad ak kòt kaban te klere syèl la nan nwit la. Anpil sitwayen vil la te sove kite vil la, genyen yo te tire gen lòt ki te tounen nan vil la lè yo te kenbe tèt ak yo. Yon milye moun vinn tonbe malad yon santèn mouri. Ki lè kochma sa a va fini? Jacksonville se te yon vil ki te anba syèj.

Pandan ke fredi ki vini nan maten mwa Novanb la tap tonbe sou kay fanmi Downing la, Maggie ki te tounen lakay li depi kèk mwa epi ki te toujou santi feblès apre li te finn troke kòn li ak lafyèv jòn la tap finn mete kouvè sou tab la lè papa Downing ak doktè Andre te pase nan pòt devan kay la epi tou dousman ak prekosyon yo te antre nan sal a manje a ak anpil soulajman yo te fè anons sa a ke moun te ap tann depi lontan. « Pa te genyen okenn nouvo ka maladi a depi pli de dijou. Li sanble ke epidemi a te fini»

Manman ak Hattie anplwaye ki te ap travay lakay la te kouri antre nan pyès la lè yo te tande nouvèl la. Manman te krye epi li te anbrase papa. Kòm yo te chita otou tab la yo remèsye Bondye de se ke li te delivre yo anba epidemi maladi lafyèv jòn la. Epidemi 1880 a te fini pa rete aprè ke fredi epòk ivè a te jele tout bagay epi elimine popilasyon moustik la. Lè yo konte a la fen epidemi a yo jwen (5000) senk mil ka maladi epi (500) senk san ka lanmò. [1]

Kòm, fè nwa te ap kouvri simityè a, mwen imajine yon zanj ki te ap pote zòm brav tankou doktè Reed ak doktè Porter sou zèl li yo ki te louvri byen gran. Mwen realize ke moun ki ap fè travay sante piblik yo se moun ki sou sou latè a ap fè travay zanj.

[1] 27 Dawou 1900, James Caroll ki te yon doktè nan lame te kite moustik ki te enfekte ak jem maladi a mode li. Li devlope yon ka grav maladi a sa ki te pèmèt doktè Walter Reed prouve ke maladi moun te pè tèlman a te trape lèke moustik ki enfekte mode moun nan. Viris lafyèv jòn la se premye viris ki nan moun ke yo te izole sa vle di mete men sou li epi ba li non viris. Doktè Porter te vinn premye ofisye lasante pou leta Florid la nan lane 1888. Nan lane 1889 yo te mete sou pye biwo ki reskonsab lisans pou travayè lasante ke yo rele" State Board of Health» Yon doktè nan lame ameriken te dekouvri moustik ki transpòte viris lafyèv jòn la ke yo rele moustik Aedes Aegypti nan lane 1900. Nan lane 1927 doktè Walter Reed te mete men sou jem ki lakòz maladi a epi li te mete anba mikroskop li jem ki lakòz lafyèv jòn la.Se akòz de dekouvèt sa a ke yo te kapab devlope yon vaksen nan lane 193. Jane Delano, yon enfimyè ki se fanmi lwen ak Franklin Delano Roosevelt se te yon volontè nan ekip resèv nan lame ameriken se te limenm ki te mete sou pye ekip enfimyè kwa rouj ameriken a, American Red Cross 1909-1912; se gras a ekip enfimyè sa a ke lè premye lagè mondyal la te eklate te genyen yon ekip uit mil enfimyè ki te pare pou ede.

How to Contact the Editors
Submit a Story
Order Additional Copies

Healthy Stories welcomes letters from its readers. Please email to HealthyStories.net or mail to:

Healthy Stories
Editorial Board
8323 NW 12th Street
Suite 214
Miami, Florida 33126

Book Prize

Healthy Stories proudly announces the Healthy Stories Book Prize. All authors or poets must submit their health related short stories, poems or recipes by February 1, 2010. Winners will be published and receive three signed copies of the book and a degree from Healthy Stories University. No reading fee. Notification by March 1, 2010.

About the Editors

MORT LAITNER

Mort Laitner has practiced law for 34 years. He commenced practicing Family Law with the Legal Aid Society of Baton Rouge, Louisiana. His next job was with Legal Services of Greater Miami where his unit handled approximately 600 cases a year.

Since 1977, he has been the chief legal counsel for the Miami-Dade County Public Health Unit, where he specializes in public health law.

Mort has taught at the University of Miami, School of Medicine, St. Thomas University, and Miami-Dade College. He has lectured throughout Florida and Georgia on public health issues.

He has handled high-profile cases which received coverage on the CBS Nightly News, Life Magazine, Money Magazine and the New York Times.

He is the author or co-author of seven books:
- *Analytical Approach For the Preparation of the Louisiana Bar Examination*
- *Les Cartes De Baton Rouge*
- *Quarantine Preparing for the Attack Small Pox: Field Exercises A how to Manual for a Beginner's Level Field Exercises*
- *SARS: A Quarantine and Isolation Manual for Severe Acute Respiratory Syndrome*
- *It is Just a Matter of Time, Recommendations that can Save Your Life*
- *Healthy Stories 2007*
- *How to Create a Public Health Film Festival*

He has produced and directed Pandemic, an avian influenza film.

Mort lives with his wife, Shelley, and has raised three sons, Jason, Travis, and Blake.

HEATHER BEATON

Heather L. Beaton was born in Miami, Florida. After graduating from Florida State University in 1999 with a degree in Political Science, Heather attended the University of Florida, Levin College of Law. She graduated with her Juris Doctorate in May 2002 with honors. Heather is a member of the Florida Bar. She currently practices law at the Miami-Dade County Health Department in the areas of contract, administrative and labor law. Heather lives with her husband, Marcos, their daughter, Kaitlyn, and a very large Boston Terrier, Blackjack.

TRACIE L. DICKERSON

Tracie L. Dickerson was born in Galveston, Texas. Tracie received her Bachelor of Science in Maritime administration form Texas A & M University, her Juris Doctor from University of Miami's School of Law and is currently pursuing a Masters in Public Health from Florida International University. Tracie is an attorney for the Miami-Dade County Health Department, specializing in Environmental Health Law. Prior to her employment with the Health Department, Tracie worked for a civil rights firm specializing in the Americans with Disabilities Act. She is a member of the Florida Bar, and is a member of the U.S. District Courts for the Southern, Middle and Northern Districts of Florida and the Southern and Northern Districts of Texas. She has also published articles in the South Florida History Magazine. Recently, Tracie gave a lecture about Healthy Stories in Orlando, Florida to the Florida Public Health Association at their yearly meeting.

ROLAND PIERRE

Roland R. Pierre was born and raised in Petion-Ville, Haiti in 1963. In Haiti, he attended "Lycée Francais" and "Lycée de Petion-Ville" where he earned his Baccalaureate First & Second Part. While he was pursuing his Baccalaureate, he attended Jamaica School of Business and the Haitiano American Institute to learn Telecommunications (Telephones Switchboard) and practice his English. He moved to US (Miami) in 1986. In 1995, He received his Associate Science (AS), and ART (AA) degrees in Computer Information Systems Analysis (CISA), and Management Information Systems (MIS) from Miami-

Dade Community College. In 1999, he graduated from Florida International University with a degree of Bachelors of Sciences in Business Administration & Management Information Systems. In 2001, he earned his Masters of Science (MSMIS) degree from Florida International University with an overall GPA of 3.56. He enjoys reading technological periodicals, playing soccer. He is a member of Florida International University Alumni.

J.D. SHINGLES
J.D. Shingles is originally from rural southwest Georgia. He moved to Miami in 1982 to work for the Grand Union Company, a grocery retailer, and Miami has since been his home. He currently works for the Miami-Dade County Health Department as a Contract Manager. He received his Bachelor's degree in Business Administration, Management from the Fort Valley State University (College). He volunteers at the Sant La Haitian Community Center as a Tax Preparer; Guardia Ad Litem; enjoys watching a good movie, mentoring, reading, fishing and traveling, whenever time permits. He is also an active member of Phi Beta Sigma Fraternity, Inc., Theta Rho Sigma Chapter.

AMY TEJIRIAN
Amy Tejirian is originally from Calgary, Alberta, Canada. She received her Bachelor of Arts degree in Communication and French from the University of California at Santa Barbara. She continued her studies at the University of Miami School of Law where she received a Juris Doctorate. Amy is a member of the both Florida and California Bars. She also has a Certificate of Public Health from the University of Florida. Amy was a kindergarten teacher for the Los Angeles Unified School District before she became an attorney, and currently, she is a contract manager for the Miami-Dade County Health Department. She speaks French and Armenian fluently. On her free time, Amy likes to travel, go the beach and attend Florida Panthers games, although her hockey favorite team is the Calgary Flames.

NINFA URDANETA

Ninfa Urdaneta is an attorney licensed to practice in the State of Florida and Venezuela. Originally from Maracaibo, Venezuela, she moved to the United States were she got married and has two adorable children. She currently works for the Legal Department/ Contracts Division for the Miami-Dade County Health Department. Through her experience in the private and governmental sectors, she has also worked for law firms, corporations and for the Venezuelan Supreme court of Justice.

FREDERICK VILLARI

Frederick Villari was born in Medfield, Massachusetts. He attended University of Miami for his undergraduate degree in Business Law and History. He continued his education at Rodger Williams University School of Law where he received his Juris Doctor. After passing the Florida Bar he went on to become an Assistant Attorney General for the Office of the Attorney General under Charlie Christ. Then he moved on in his legal career to the Miami-Dade County State Attorney's Office under Katherine Fernandez-Rundle and served as an Assistant State Attorney. He has finally found his home and family working for the Miami-Dade County Health Department. He is currently licensed to practice law in Florida and the District of Columbia. Frederick is happily married to Francesca and they have a beautiful baby boy named Frederick Joseph Villari, IV.

Praise for Healthy Stories

"Healthy Stories is a fascinating compilation of stories written by those who have had the experience of providing Public Health to those in our care. These stories are compelling and powerful vignettes meant to both enlighten and inspire."

Florida Public Health Association, *Green Cove Springs, FL*

"I thoroughly enjoyed Healthy Stories particularly The Band-Aid. It clearly reminds us that advocacy is not just a nine-to-five job."

Dr. Alexis Powell, M.D., *Miami, FL Assistant Clinical Professor University of Miami Department of Medicine, Division of Infectious Diseases*

"Healthy Stories is like a 'lighthouse' to guide you through the waves of life."

Monroe Edelstein, *Dade City, FL*

"I really enjoyed reading Healthy Stories – it made what we do everyday so much more real – not just the dry "facts of the case" we lawyers get caught up in. Thanks for giving me a new perspective."

Janine B. Myrick, *JD, Tallahassee, FL Director, Division of Health Access and Tobacco Florida Department of Health*

"I read a wonderful article about Healthy Stories. I would love to order print copies for our breast cancer program coordinators in Michigan for their work."

Julie I. Williams, *MPH, Detroit, MI*
Wayne State University
The National Cancer Institute's Cancer
Information Service at Karmanos Cancer Institute

"Great story, very visual, wonder if it could be dramatized and video-taped (like a 30 second commercial) and posted on our website."

Rene J. Borroto-Ponce, *Miami, FL Concerning Signs*

"I have read Healthy Stories to the students in my Essentials of Public Health Practice class and they have been both entertained and educated."

Judy Perkin, DrPH, RD, CHES, *Professor*
Brooks College of Health, University of North Florida